Praise for *Hair Story*

"An engaging look at what has become a major status symbol among African-Americans . . . an impressive work of cultural history."

—*BookPage*

"*Hair Story* presents an absorbing rendition of American history told through Black hair. In prose that is both humorous and haunting, the authors manage to bring vividly to life a subject most would consider inconsequential. After reading this comprehensive tale, people will walk away with a whole new appreciation for Black hair and all of its wonder and power!"

—Lloyd Boston, author of the bestselling
Men of Color: Fashion, History, and Fundamentals

"From antiquity to the present day, Black hair has been both ornamentation and a medium of artistic expression. At the same time, its changing political and cultural values have often mirrored the current social climate. *Hair Story*, in documenting our natural hair's beauty and capacity for communication, brings to life and infuses with historical relevance this unique slice of Americana."

—Harriette Cole,
author of *Jumping the Broom* and *How to Be*

"Keen historical insight with pop-cultural anecdotes."

—*Entertainment Weekly*

"A comprehensive and colorful look at a very touchy subject."

—*Essence*

"As far as neatly and efficiently chronicling African-Americans and the importance of their hair, *Hair Story* gets to the root of things."

—Philadelphiaweekly.com

"{An} entertaining and concise survey . . . a book that successfully balances popular appeal with historical accuracy."

—Publishers Weekly

"Taps into the art and history of how Black hair is perceived in America in a way that will no doubt be relevant for generations to come."

—The Source

St. Martin's Griffin

New York

HAIR STORY

Revised Edition

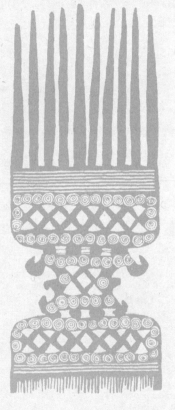

Untangling

the Roots

of Black Hair

in America

AYANA D. BYRD AND LORI L. THARPS

For Dayvon Baldwin, Samuel R. Byrd,

Manuel J. Malia, Quincy and

Morris Tharps, and Stephanie Williams

HAIR STORY. Copyright © 2001, 2014 by Ayana D. Byrd and Lori L. Tharps. All rights reserved. Printed in the United States of America. For information, address St. Martin's Press, 175 Fifth Avenue, New York, N.Y. 10010.

www.stmartins.com

THE LIBRARY OF CONGRESS CATALOGING-IN-PUBLICATION DATA IS AVAILABLE UPON REQUEST.

ISBN 978-1-250-04657-4 (trade paperback)
ISBN 978-1-4668-4682-1 (e-book)

St. Martin's Griffin books may be purchased for educational, business, or promotional use. For information on bulk purchases, please contact Macmillan Corporate and Premium Sales Department at 1-800-221-7945, extension 5442, or write specialmarkets@macmillan.com.

10 9 8 7 6 5 4 3 2

Contents

Acknowledgments

This could not have happened without the support and love of our families and friends, who are too numerous to list by name but who each individually contributed in their own special, much-needed ways. A special thanks to the Tharps, Price-Williams, Byrd, Malia-Camacho, Winston-Porter-Pope, and Baldwin-Taylor families.

The inspiration for *Hair Story* began in a Belgian beauty salon and in a living room in Morocco. The idea was developed in two separate projects at Barnard College and Columbia University's Graduate School of Journalism. Much sincere thanks and appreciation to those professors who encouraged us to take the next step—Helen Benedict, Lynn Chancer, Natalie Kampen, and Les Lessinger.

Special thanks to Dave Bry and the Vibe Research Department for bringing us together and to our diner in Brooklyn Heights for nourishing us (literally) as we took the first slow, faltering steps of putting thoughts to paper; Marie Brown, the most laid-back literary agent, who not only sold us on the idea that we could do this but then convinced the rest of the world. To Glenda Howard and the people at St. Martin's Press, who have shared our excitement and enthusiasm and helped fine-tune the vision behind this book.

It took about one week of writing to realize that this would only be possible with the assistance of others. We'd especially like to thank Ernest Montgomery, photo editor extraordinaire, for being both brilliant and cost-effective; Samuel R. Byrd for his artistic genius and speed; Asali Solomon for catching all of our most obvious mistakes and making us sound literate; Dana King, our amazing researcher, for her contributions, suggestions, and belief in our project; Miko McGinty for all your design directives and creative eye; Manuel Malia for his eagle-eye copyediting and constructive criticism; Gael Levin, Karen R. Good, and Christian Bernard for their computers and friendly encouragement; Tesha McCord for her legal advice; to Alfonso Smith for the photos; April Garrett for her bottomless Rolodex; Andrew Gillings for the access code; Kofi Taha for, as always, stepping in and saving the day; Godwin Mensah for technical support and a glimpse into Ghana; Fallon Scoggins and Mia Herndon; all of the women and men who shared their hair stories, providing us with many of the anecdotes in the book; to the friendly security guard at *Entertainment Weekly* who kept us safe after hours.

Thanks to the Solomon family—Rochell and James for giving up a Sunday football game to recount their hair stories and Akiba for photo-documenting the outrageousness of her eighties hair; A'Lelia Bundles for always cheerfully providing the answers to our endless barrage of questions; Nat "The Bush Doctor" Mathis for sharing his life with us over a Chinese dinner and for proving to the world that Black hair is worth immortalizing; Carolivia Herron, bell hooks, Dr. Cheryl Ajirotutu, Harriette Cole, Lloyd Boston, Geri Duncan Jones and the AHBAI, Bernice Calvin, Marcia Gillespie, and Glynn Jackson for their insights into the world of Black hair culture; the Indiana Historical Society and New York's Schomburg Research Library; Willie Morrow for just being himself; the supportive staffs of *Entertainment Weekly, Vibe,* and *Rolling Stone* magazines; Dawn Baskerville at *InStyle;* MOET (Men of *Ego Trip*); Santi White for always understanding that sometimes this book needed to come first; and Shanita (just because).

Inspiration from the spirits and life's work of Madam C. J. Walker and Annie Turnbo Malone; Assata Shakur and Angela Davis; and Lisa Jones, who first brought the "hair beat" to the masses. And to Florence Price, whose outrageous statements and no-holds-barred opinions of what hair should look like have been a constant inspiration and an almost constant cross to bear.

Authors' Note

We often like to tell the story of how *Hair Story* came to be. Back in 1997, we were both fact-checkers at *Vibe* magazine, and it's an understatement to say we worked long hours. So, one night around midnight, our supervisor asked if we were aware that the two of us shared an academic-y fascination with Black hair. Ayana had created a two-year-long honor's program project on Black hair, Black women, and beauty ideals as an undergraduate, and Lori wrote her masters thesis on the politics, business, and history of Black hair. Suddenly shaken from our sleepy delirium, we started to talk about hair and realized we'd each found a kindred spirit in the other, one who saw the need for serious scholarship on the topic. For the next few weeks we shared our personal hair stories, learning that we had much in common.

Growing up in Philadelphia and Milwaukee and then in our lives as transplanted New Yorkers, we knew Black people had hair on the brain as much as we did. And that other ethnic groups had questions and ideas—both good and bad—about what they saw on Black people's heads. We were teenagers when the newspapers were filled with stories of African-American women who were losing their jobs on account of their braided hairstyles; we both came of age when the Jheri Curl was all the rage and knew people who rocked the style way past its heyday; and even though we grew up in totally different areas of the country, we both heard whispers about "good hair" and knew what it meant if you didn't have it.

We also both realized that as much as we shared this common hair story, non-Black people had no idea what we were talking about. It was perplexing that something so familiar to us and other Black people was so foreign to our coworkers, friends, and others of a different race. We wanted to not only document this incredibly pertinent and fascinating slice of Black American history, but also to give non-Black Americans a resource to understand an aspect of American culture that they saw every day but rarely understood.

So, we decided to do just that. We took the sociological aspects of Ayana's college project, merged them with the historical focus of Lori's, and got on planes, trains, and automobiles to interview people, visit important places where hair history was made, and basically live on the ground floor of the library at the Schomburg Center for Research in Black Culture in Harlem. We felt like detectives, piecing together primary sources and finding experts in the field of Black hair to provide context to the story we were trying to tell. This was before the Internet was considered reliable, so we were lucky enough to have face-to-face conversations, sit in barbershops, flip through family photo albums, and actually touch the artifacts collected by the Madam C. J. Walker estate when we visited her archives in Indianapolis. It was Black hair heaven for two people as obsessed as we were and validation that this was a story that needed to be collected, structured, put into some context, and shared.

So today, thirteen years after *Hair Story*'s original release, it seems like everyone is thinking and talking about hair—and not just in their kitchens, but out loud in public, on the Internet, and in classrooms, documentaries, and books. And it's no longer just Black people taking part in the conversation. Mainstream media outlets—from HBO to *The New York Times*—have covered the topic of hair on screen and in print. White movie stars with adopted Black children have become unintentional ambassadors, bringing Black hair culture to a wider mainstream audience; international artists have used Black hair as a theme in their work; academic institutions hold panels on the topic and offer courses covering Black hair politics; and talk show hosts looking to boost their ratings have examined the divisive topic of "good hair" on the air.

It's wrong to think that Black hair is such a popular topic because it's a painful one. We have always believed that even though Black people might have a lot of convoluted feelings about their hair, and non-Black people might be confused when confronted with our kinks and curls, there is also a lot of beauty and pride in the subject. In addition, there is a lot of comfort and meaning in Black hair culture. The word "culture" often gets misused and overused, but with Black hair there is a real culture, in the way that anthropologists would define it: the learned patterns of behavior and thought that assist a group in adapting to its environment and include ritual, language, memory, and evolution. We wrote *Hair Story* to define and celebrate that culture—to untangle the rituals, language, and memories from an American history that ignored its existence. And since history is a collection of yesterdays, this Black hair history continues, and we are honored and excited to continue to tell the tale.

—AYANA D. BYRD AND LORI L. THARPS

1

Black Hair in Bondage:
1400–1899

The Story Starts in Africa

The story of Black people's hair begins where everything began—in Africa. Not surprisingly, the birthplace of both astronomy and alchemy also gave rise to a people in perfect harmony with their environment. Indeed the dense, spiraling curls of African hair demonstrate evolutionary genius. Like natural air-conditioning, this frizzy, kinky hair insulates the head from the brutal intensity of the sun's rays. Of course there is not one single type of African hair, just as there is not one single type of African. The variety of hair textures from western Africa alone ranges from the deep ebony, kinky curls of the Mandingos to the loosely curled, flowing locs of the Ashanti. The one constant Africans share when it comes to hair is the social and cultural significance intrinsic to each beautiful strand.

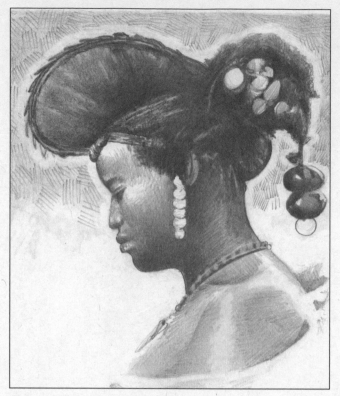

© Samuel R. Byrd.

In the early fifteenth century, hair functioned as a carrier of messages in most West African societies. The citizens of these societies—including the Wolof, Mende, Mandingo, and Yoruba—were the people who filled the slave ships that sailed to the "New World." Within these cultures, hair was an integral part of a complex language system. Ever since African civilizations bloomed, hairstyles have been used to indicate a person's marital status, age, religion, ethnic identity, wealth, and rank within the community. In some cultures a person's surname could be ascertained simply by examining the hair because each clan had its own unique hairstyle. The hairstyle also served as an indicator of a person's geographic origins. The Kuramo people of Nigeria, for example, were recognized by their unique coiffure—a shaved head with a single tuft of hair left on top. In the Wolof culture of Senegal, young girls who were not of marrying age partially shaved their heads to emphasize their unavailability for courting. Likewise a recently widowed woman stopped attending to her hair for a specified mourning period because she was not meant to look beautiful to other men, and an unkempt coiffure in almost every West African culture was anathema to the opposite sex. Nigerian housewives living in a polygamous society created a hairstyle intended to taunt their husband's other wives. The style was known as *kohin-sorogun* ("turn your back to the jealous rival wife") and was meant to be seen from behind. In ancient times, if a Wolof man wore his hair in a particular braided hairdo it meant he was preparing to go to war and therefore prepared to die. Such a man would then tell his wife she should not comb her hair because in a matter of hours she could become a widow. Traditionally the leaders of a community—men and women—showcased the most ornate hairstyles, and only royalty or the equivalent would be expected to wear a hat or headpiece. "The common people go bareheaded," wrote French anthropologist Marie Armand Pascal

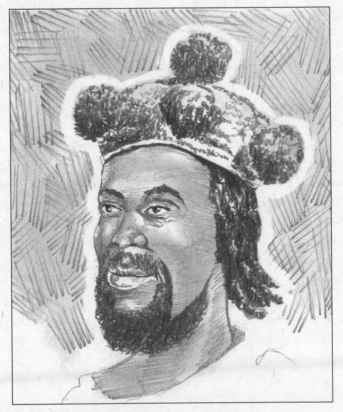

© Samuel R. Byrd.

d'Avezac-Macaya when describing the Ijebu people living near the coast of Guinea. "As for the king, his headdress is raised up in the form of a tiara of great richness. It is made of coral beads mounted close together on a background of crimson leather; at the crest is a tuft or tassel of gold braid."

While the social significance of the hair was weighty for African people, the aesthetic aspects were just as important. "West African communities admire a fine head of long, thick hair on a woman. A woman with long, thick hair demonstrates the life-force, the multiplying power of profusion, prosperity, a 'green thumb' for raising bountiful farms and many healthy children," wrote Sylvia Ardyn Boone, an anthropologist specializing in the Mende culture of Sierra Leone. According to Boone, "big hair, plenty of hair, much hair," were the qualities every woman wanted. But there was more to being beautiful than simply having a lot of hair. It had to be clean, neat, and arranged in a specific style—usually a braided design—to conform to tradition. A particular style could be intended to attract someone of the opposite sex or signal a religious ritual. In Nigeria, if a woman left her hair undone, it was a signal that something was wrong. The woman was either bereaved, depressed, or "habitually dirty." To the Mende, unkempt, "neglected," or "messy" hair implied that a woman either had loose morals or was insane. Mohamed Mbodj, associate professor of history at Columbia University and a native of Dakar, Senegal, says that Boone's description of the Mende's beauty ideal regarding hair also applied to the Senegalese: "[Wolof] women liked to have their hair shiny and long. And you didn't cut it, you arranged it." Mbodj also concurs that an unkempt or disheveled hairdo was often interpreted as a sign of dementia. Men, too, were always expected to keep their locs neat and tidy, whether they wore a short style or an elaborate creation.

The hair's value and worth were heightened by its spiritual qualities. Both male and female devotees of certain Yoruba gods and goddesses were required to keep their hair braided in a specific style. "The hair is the most elevated point of your body, which means it is the closest to the divine," Mbodj explains as an indication of the power the hair holds. Because the hair is the closest thing to the heavens, communication from the gods and spirits was thought to pass through the hair to get to the soul. Mbodj also notes that spells could be cast or harm could be brought to another person by acquiring a single strand of their hair. Wolof tradition says that women had the power to make men crazy for them by calling on the power of the

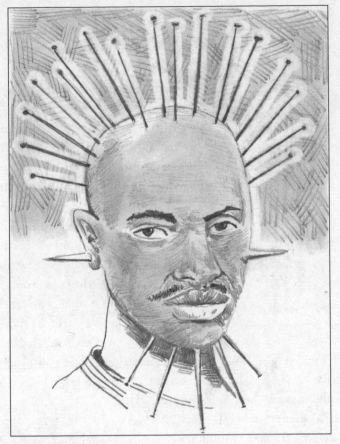

© Samuel R. Byrd.

genies and spirits in the hair. The hair was thought to be so powerful that medicine men in Cameroon used human hair to adorn the vessels and containers in which they carried their healing potions as a means of protection and added potency.

Because a person's spirit supposedly nestled in the hair, the hairdresser always held a special place in community life. The hairdresser was often considered the most trustworthy individual in society. The complicated and time-consuming task of hair grooming included washing, combing, oiling, braiding, twisting, and/or decorating the hair with any number of adornments including cloth, beads, and shells. The process could last several hours, sometimes several days. Often the only tools the hairdresser used were a hand-carved wooden comb (specifically designed with long

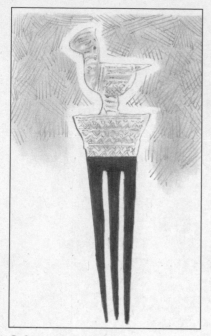

© Samuel R. Byrd.

teeth and rounded tips to remove tangles and knots without causing excessive pain), palm oil, and years of creative know-how. In some cultures the hair was groomed by a family member because only a relative could be trusted with such an important task. In the Yoruba tradition, all women were taught how to braid, but any young girl who showed talent in the art of hairdressing was encouraged to become a "master," assuming responsibility for the entire community's coiffures. Before a "master" died, she would pass on her box of hairdressing tools to a successor within the family during a sacred ceremony. For the Mende, offering to braid someone else's hair was a way of asking them to be your friend. Boone writes, "Hair-braiding sessions are a time

of shared confidences and laughter; the circle of women who do each other's hair are friends bound together in a fellowship." In communities in both Ghana and Senegal, women were not allowed to groom men's hair and vice versa because of the social taboo that restricted interactions between the sexes. In addition, the only people allowed to work on hair, Mbodj says, were the griots and the ironworkers. "Anybody who is working at creating life with dead material, like melting iron and making it into something new," Mbodj explains, "those are the people who have the exclusive right to

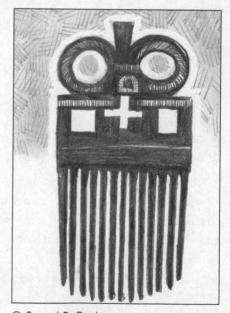

© Samuel R. Byrd.

work on people's hair." When Wolof children were born they would inherit a hairdresser, based on familial relationships, who would remain in their service for life.

Clearly hair has never been a purely cosmetic attribute for the West African people. Its social, aesthetic, and spiritual significance has been intrinsic to their sense of self for thousands of years. It is a testament to the strength of these African cultures that the same rituals and beliefs regarding the hair remain in traditional societies today.

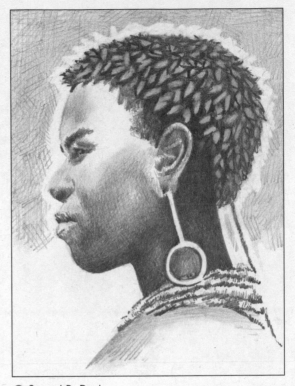

© Samuel R. Byrd.

Although Africans were neither the first nor the only people who elevated the significance of hair in their cultural milieu, when Europeans first came in contact with the African natives in the fifteenth century they were astounded by the complexity of style, texture, and adornment of Black hair.

The Slave Trade

When the first Europeans began exploring the western coast of Africa around 1444, they were chasing fantasies of unclaimed riches. Instead of finding virgin territory flush with golden treasure, however, the European travelers discovered thriving African nations and new trading partners. For almost a hundred years thereafter, the Europeans enjoyed a cordial trading relationship with the Africans, exchanging weapons, textiles, liquor, and

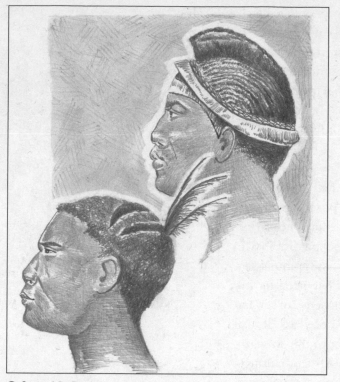

© Samuel R. Byrd.

shiny baubles for gold, ivory, and sometimes even a small number of human slaves, who would be taken to the European continent and sold. This was a productive time for European exploration of the West African coast, and many men wrote about the majestic Africans they met along the way. Not only were these White men dazzled by the fantastic agricultural products the Africans were growing, such as corn, peanuts, and tobacco, and the vibrant indigo dyes used to color clothing and materials, they were also duly impressed by the extraordinary African hairstyles. "The Senegal blacks [have] their hair either curled or long and lank, and piled up on their head in the shape of a pointed hat," wrote French explorer Jean Barbot. The Qua-qua, on the other hand, "wear long locs of hair, plaited and twisted, which they daub with palm oil and red earth. This hair is the hair of their wives, which they cut off and tie it this way, end to end, and fix it on their heads; some let it hang down, others turn it up!" Even though some of the Africans with whom the Europeans came in contact wore very little in the way of clothing—sometimes only a well-placed loincloth—the hairstyles were often elaborate works of art, showcasing braids, plaits, patterns shaved into the scalp, and any combination of shells, flowers, beads, or strips of material woven into the hair. "The king in Sierra Lionna [sic]," recalled Barbot, had "on his head a sort of cap made of straw in the shape of a mitre, decorated with goats [sic] horns, small porcupine tails and other trifles . . . his hair was tied up one on each side in such a way that from a distance the points could have been taken for the horns of some animal." One Dutch explorer, while in the country of Benin, noted sixteen different hairstyles, each one indicating a combination of gender and status within the community. Unstyled and unkempt hair was largely unseen, as were scarves or headwraps. Clearly nothing was meant to cover the African people's crowning glory.

By the beginning of the sixteenth century the Spanish, Dutch, Portuguese, British, and French had begun conquering new territories in North America, South America, and the islands of the Caribbean. These enthusiastic conquistadors found themselves in the unprofitable position of occupying entire islands and countries, unable to work the verdant lands to capacity. Realizing the need for an imported labor force, the Europeans reassessed their West African trading partners. Since the Africans themselves were willing to trade in human cargo, the Europeans sought to exploit the situation. It was at this point that the African slave trade began in earnest. No longer content to take a few slaves back to Europe for a meager

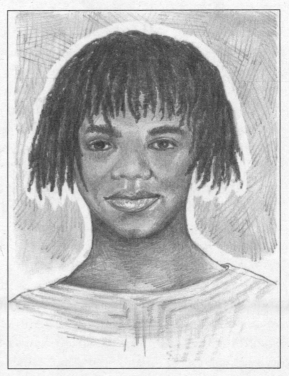

© Samuel R. Byrd.

profit, the newly dubbed slave traders made several voyages a year to the area they baptized the Slave Coast (formerly known as the Gold Coast). There they acquired anywhere from one hundred to three hundred bodies at a time, which were then sold for a handsome profit to eager colonists in their new homelands. To keep up with the demand and to take advantage of the Europeans' seemingly inexhaustible wealth, the stronger West African city-states increased their raids on the smaller inland nations seeking slaves to sell. Family members began to sell their own relatives, and debtors, social outcasts, and prisoners of war became unfortunate pawns in the slave trade.

For nearly four hundred years, an estimated twenty million men, women, and children were forcibly removed from their homes and dragged in chains to the slave markets on that infamous coast that stretched for three thousand miles from Senegal to Angola. The captives were then sold to European and Arabian slave traders. Most of the slaves were between the ages of ten and twenty-four, and the majority of them hailed from Western and West Central Africa. The citizens of countries such as Senegal, Gambia, Sierra Leone, Ghana, and Nigeria were highly sought after because of their specialized skills in agriculture, pottery, jewelry making, cotton weaving, and woodworking. One of the first things the slave traders did to their new cargo was shave their heads if they had not already been shorn by their captors. The "highest indignity," wrote Ayuba Suleiman Diallo, a member of a prominent West African family who was kidnapped and forced into slavery, was when his Mandingo assailants shaved his head and beard to make him appear as if he were a prisoner taken in war.

Given the importance of the hair to an African, having the head shaved was an unspeakable crime. Indeed, offers Frank Herreman, director of exhibitions at New York's Museum for African Art and specialist in African hairstyles, "a shaved head can be interpreted as taking away someone's identity." Presumably the slave traders shaved the heads of their new slaves for what they considered sanitary reasons, but the effect was much more insidious. The shaved head was the first step the Europeans took to erase the slave's culture and alter the relationship between the African and his or her hair. Separating individuals from family and community on the slave ships during the middle passage furthered their alienation from everything they had ever known. Arriving without their signature hairstyles, Mandingos, Fulanis, Ibos, and Ashantis entered the New World, just as the Europeans intended, like anonymous chattel.

The first African slaves, a group of only twenty, were brought to British North America in 1619 (long after the first slaves arrived in the Caribbean). They arrived in Jamestown at the same time the first White women set foot in the new colony. As the British had neither social nor political experience in dealing with slaves, the first African captives were contracted to work under the same terms as the White indentured servants arriving mainly from England, Scotland, and Ireland. After working a specified number of years, the Africans were allowed to buy their freedom and become contributing members of society. In addition, owing to the scant number of White females, some European men sought Native American and Black women for companionship and eventually had children with them. "These laboring [European] people themselves had been aliens at home, they were aliens in America and they were not so steeped in the color code," historian Joel Williamson wrote about cross-cultural coupling in the early days of the British colonies. Because English law at the time declared that children inherited the status of their fathers, any mixed child with a European father was considered free at birth. Most mixed-race individuals, asserts Williamson, were the offspring of White "servants" and Black people. The result was an early North America infused with a medley of skin colors, hair textures, and interracial identities.

As the years passed, however, indentured servitude for Blacks evolved into a race-based institution called slavery. One by one, laws were put into effect that systematically took away the rights of Black people, as the British embraced the economic advantage of slavery. In 1641 Massachusetts became the first English colony to legalize slavery. In 1662 Virginia courts reversed the status-of-the-father clause so that children inherited the status of their mother. Now children born to slaves were also condemned to slavery. And finally in 1670 Virginia declared that baptism did not alter a person's condition as regards to the state of bondage or freedom. In other words, even Africans who converted to Christianity were not saved from the chains of eternal servitude. The tide had turned and the deck was stacked against Black people, but still Blacks, Whites, and Native Americans continued to procreate (often by force) and populate the land with mixed-race individuals who often fell between the lines of the law. There were a few mulattoes during this ambiguous colonial period, in fact, who were able to prosper and even owned slaves themselves. By the early 1700s, however, any person with proven African ancestry—even a single relative from one hundred years back—was considered Black and therefore eligible to be enslaved. The thirty or so years when Black Africans had been realistically able to work for freedom quickly faded from memory, and Black people arriving on the shores of a hostile land faced a life without hope for a future.

Black Hair in Bondage

The primary need for slaves in British North America was to work on the massive plantations in the mid-Atlantic and southern states. While some slaves were purchased by farmers and tradesmen living in the North, the vast majority of Black Africans arrived to find themselves sold to southern plantation owners trying their hand at growing cotton, tobacco, and/or rice. Slave owners were very interested in the Africans' agricultural expertise, specifically at growing rice, but for the most part showed no inclination to respect the Africans' humanity or culture. Slave owners wanted maximum output from each slave, often choosing to work them to death in a matter of years rather than show them a bit of compassion. The slaves were expected to work in the fields under a grueling sun for twelve to fifteen hours a day, seven days a week. The single meal of the day might consist of dry cornbread smeared with pork grease and some type of overcooked vegetable. Punishments for insolence, slowing down, or rebellion included whippings with a cat-o'-nine-tails, sadistic torture, and amputations of digits and limbs.

Given these inhumane and unhealthy conditions, the Africans had neither the time nor the inclination to care much about their appearance, including their hair. Moreover, treasured African combs were nowhere to be found in the New World, so the once long, thick, and healthy tresses of both women and men became tangled and matted. Out of desperation for a tool to replace the African combs, the slaves began using a sheep fleece carding tool to untangle their hair. Interestingly, there appears to be no record of slaves making new combs specifically designed for their kinky hair. "We carded our hair cuz we never had no combs, but the cards they worked better," recalled former slave Jane Morgan in an interview with a government worker from the Work Projects Administration (WPA). "We used the cards to card wool with also, and we just wet our hair and then card it. The cards had wooden handles and strong steel wire teeth," Morgan recalled. Scalp diseases like ringworm became pervasive among the slave population, as did lice infestations. When an outbreak of ringworm occurred, slaves commonly tied a rag around their heads to cover the unsightly scabs left by the affliction, and a worse infection would then ensue, creating a vicious cycle of hair problems, breakage, and patchy baldness. Whereas in Africa, women could spend hours a day grooming their hair and arranging it in traditional styles, on the plantations they used scarves or kerchiefs fashioned from coarse fabric scraps provided by stingy masters to keep their hair well hidden. Partly as protection from the scorching sun and hovering flies and partly out of shame for the now unsightly hair, the head rag became ubiquitous in slave culture.

A crucial determinant of how slaves wore their hair was their work assignment. For the slaves who toiled in the fields and lived in separate slave quarters, the women wore head rags and the men took to shaving their heads, wearing straw hats, or using animal shears to cut their hair short. On the other hand, the slaves who experienced a closer relationship with the White population—laundresses, barbers, cooks, nursemaids, housekeepers, chauffeurs, valets—often styled their hair in an imitation of their White owners. For example, in the eighteenth century it was fashionable for White men of the upper class to wear wigs. As a result, some Black slaves took to wearing wigs as well; others shaped and styled their own hair to look like a wig. The slaves who worked inside the plantation houses were required to present a neat and tidy appearance or risk the wrath of the master, so men and women often wore tight braids, plaits, and cornrows (made by sectioning the hair and braiding it flat to the scalp). The braid patterns were commonly based on African tradition and styles. Other styles Blacks wore proved to be an amalgam of traditional African styles, European trends, and even Native American practices. One runaway slave was described as having "the Top of his head Shaved, and he combs it back like a woman." It was not uncommon to see Black men with long ponytails (called "queues") and partially shaved heads and Black women with their hair parted down the middle and brushed into a version of a European style.

In this new land dominated by pale skin and straight hair, African hair was deemed wholly unattractive and inferior by the Europeans. Many White people went so far as to insist that Blacks did not have real hair, preferring to classify it in a derogatory manner as "wool." Descriptions of Black hair in the early 1700s—in runaway slave advertisements, slave auction posters, and even the daily newspapers—use this classification, almost as if by likening the hair to an animal's, Whites would be validated in their inhumane treatment of Blacks. "Before you can subjugate or oppress people you must relabel them as subhuman," declares Joy DeGruy Leary, a mental health therapist and Ph.D. studying the transgenerational trauma African-Americans suffered because of slavery. Once the feminine beauty ideal was characterized as requiring "long straight hair, with fine features," says DeGruy Leary, White slave owners sought to pathologize African features like dark skin and kinky hair to further demoralize the slaves, especially the women. Aided by the scientific community, which had officially relegated dark-skinned, "woolly"-haired people to the bottom of the evolutionary ladder, the slave owners' brainwashing took root. "Black women began to perceive themselves as ugly and inferior," DeGruy Leary says. "And if you believe you're inferior, then you're much easier to control." On the part of the slave owners, she adds, this brainwashing was not accidental, but deliberate. When the slave women internalized the slave owner's racist rhetoric, which was almost inevitable, it wasn't long before they passed the pathology on to their sons, daughters, and future generations.

Even though slave masters did their best to break the spirit of the Black people, the hair refused to relinquish its unique character, and some slaves consciously chose not to hide it. Runaway slave notices posted in the 1700s, for example, make mention of flamboyant hairstyles that belie any sense of shame or inferiority. The following hair descriptions of runaways were used in an East Coast newspaper at the time: "strong bearded and hair longer than Negroes commonly have," "a very good head of hair," "a short chubby fellow with extraordinary bushy hair," "A Negro man his hair on the top with a tupee foretop," "his hair is cut short on his crown but curls around his neck," "his hair grows down his forehead and is bare on the temple." Meanwhile a female runaway, Kate, from South Carolina, had "bushy hair, which she is apt to keep uncombed." Even though unkempt hair went against the African aesthetic, some historians suggest that such unconventional styles were a way for Black people to assert their individuality and humanity in the repressive slave culture. "Hair that was worn long and bushy," argue Shane and Graham White, authors of *Stylin': Afri-*

can American Expressive Culture from Its Beginnings to the Zoot Suit, "empha-sized and even flaunted its distinctive texture [and] may have been an affirmation of difference and even of defiance, an attempt to revalorize a biological characteristic that White racism had sought to devalue." With a steady stream of Africans entering the slave population, the meaning and significance of traditional hairstyles was not easily forgotten. It has even been suggested that in the first century of North American slavery, some of the more unique styles worn by men, like the combination ponytail and shaved head hairdos, were used in place of ritual scarification or for rite-of-passage ceremonies. White and White suggest that "the elaborate and distinctive styling of male hair may well have served as a form of substitute bodily decoration that still marked these young men off but seemed rather more attuned to their new circumstances as American slaves."

By the time the transatlantic slave trade was outlawed in North America in 1808, a distinct Black American culture had developed. As described by authors Charles Johnson and Patricia Smith in *Africans in America,* "This new culture became an intriguing mixture of African traditions and those developed in the Americas as a means for survival. Blacks from different parts of Africa combined their beliefs, their music, and their languages while borrowing from the European culture to create a commonality." Though slaves could still be bought and sold, they were no longer being imported from Africa. With this peculiar institution of domestic slavery firmly en-trenched in American society, a plantation owner was often judged not just by the quantity of his slaves but the quality as well. Sickly and unsightly slaves were both a bad reflection on the slave owner and a difficult commod-ity to sell. So while life did not suddenly become pleasant and amicable for the slaves, they were allocated some time for personal grooming. It was around this time that many slave owners began to allow their slaves to "rest" on Sundays in order to attend church and observe the Sabbath.

Because this was the only day when there was time to devote to one-self, Sundays became the designated day for doing hair. "The only time the slaves had to comb their hair was on Sunday," former slave James Wil-liams told a WPA interviewer. "They would comb and roll each other's hair and the men cut each other's hair. That all the time they got." Another former slave, Charlie Hudson, had similar memories. "Sundays the old folks stayed home and looked one another's heads over for nits and lice.

Then, the womans wrapped each other's hair so it would stay fixed till the next Sunday." In Natchez, Mississippi, a White New England traveler described the following Sunday morning church preparations in the slave quarters. "In every cabin the men are shaving and dressing—the women, arrayed in their gay muslins, are arranging their frizzy hair, in which they take no little pride." All week the hair might be hidden under a scarf, but for church on Sundays the hair would be combed out and styled. "In them days all the darky wommens wore they hair in string 'cept when they tended church or a wedding," recalled former slave Gus Fester. Amos Lincoln added, "All week they wear they hair all roll with cotton that they unfold off the cotton ball. Sunday come they comb out they hair fine. They want it nice and natural curly." Besides serving as the spiritual renewal for the week, church also became the place for the slaves to exchange hair remedies and secrets.

HOMEMADE HAIR CARE

After two centuries in bondage, a unique homegrown system of Black hair care had developed. Over the years, the goal of grooming the hair had morphed from the elaborate and symbolic designs of Africa into an imitation of White styles adapted to Black kinks and curls. Both women and men were interested in straightening their hair because straight European hair was held up as the beauty ideal. There existed neither a public nor a private forum where Black hair was celebrated in America. And without the influx of Africans to the slave population, it was difficult for Blacks born and raised in captivity to take pride in their kinky locs.

Without the combs, herbal ointments, and palm oil used in Africa for hairdressing, the slaves were forced to use common Western household products and equipment to achieve certain styles. Instead of palm oil, the slaves took to using oil-based products like bacon grease and butter to condition and soften the hair, prepare it for straightening, and make it shine. Cornmeal and kerosene were used as scalp cleaners, and coffee became a natural dye for women. Several methods of straightening the hair were concocted by ingenious Blacks who were short on commercial products. Men would slick axle grease meant for wagon wheels over their hair for a combination dye job and straightener. Women would slather the hair with butter, bacon fat, or goose grease and then use a butter knife heated in a can over a fire as a crude curling iron. Sometimes a piece of cloth warmed over a flame would be pulled across the head and worn for a short while to stretch the curls out. Women also wrapped their hair in strings, strips of nylon, cotton, or eel skin to decrease the kink and leave looser curls. Some slave mothers took to wrapping their children's hair to start "training" it to go straight as early as infancy. The most mordant device used to straighten the hair was lye, mixed with potatoes to decrease its caustic nature. This creamy concoction was smeared on the hair and the lye would straighten the curls. Unfortunately, it could also eat the skin right off a person's head.

"Good" and "Bad" Hair

The quest for straight hair was often a torturous obsession for the slaves, but it was not just about conforming to the prevailing fashions of the day. Straight hair translated to economic opportunity and social advantage. Because many of the more than one hundred thousand free Blacks in nineteenth-century America were the mulatto offspring of the first African arrivals and their European companions, lighter skin and loosely curled hair would often signify free status. In fact, many light-complected slaves tried to pass themselves off as free, hoping their European features would be enough to convince bounty hunters that they belonged to that privileged class. "A mulatto wench is very well featured all but her nose and lips which are thick and flat," read an announcement for a runaway in the *New York Gazette*. "Has long black curld [sic] hair, may pass for a free person." Curiously, the hair was considered the most telling feature of Negro status, more than the color of the skin. Even though some slaves (many of them products of interracial coupling between slave and master) had skin as light as many Whites, the rule of thumb was that if the hair showed just a little bit of kinkiness, a person would be unable to pass as White. Essentially, the hair acted as the true test of Blackness, which is why some male slaves opted to shave their heads to try to get rid of the genetic evidence of their ancestry when attempting to escape to freedom. Consider this description of a runaway posted in the *New York Weekly Journal:* "A mulatto man, aged 23, pretty fair with his head commonly shaved in order to make himself pass for a white man."

Straight hair was not only about freedom for a slave. Those slaves living on plantations soon realized that lighter-skinned Blacks with straighter hair worked inside the plantation houses performing less backbreaking labor than the slaves relegated to the fields. The slaves who worked in the house also had access to hand-me-down clothes, better food, education, and sometimes even the promise of freedom upon the master's death. The reason the lighter-skinned, straighter-haired slaves were chosen for domestic service has a lot to do with the fact that many of these mixed-race slaves were the offspring of the master or his son. Noted American slave historian Kenneth M. Stamp confirmed that "unmarried slaveholders and the young males who grew up in slave holding families, some bearing the South's most distinguished names, played a major role in [miscegenation]. Indeed, given their easy access to female slaves, it seems probable that miscegenation was more common among them than among any other group." Slaves with light skin and straight hair also might have been favored because it was easier for the White masters and mistresses to have people with familiar physical features waiting on them in their own home. And, of course, the "exotic"-looking mulatto female slaves were often chosen to work in the master's house because he had every intention of making her his sex slave. "Slaves selected for their grace, beauty and light skins were shipped to the fancy-girl markets of New Orleans and other cities. Some ended up in bordellos, but the majority became the mistresses of wealthy planters, gamblers, or businessmen," wrote historian Dorothy Sterling in *We Are Your Sisters*. Coincidentally, as these female slaves with long, loosely curled hair entered the plantation houses, the plantation wives instituted a new form of punishment for them. The jealous mistress of the manor often shaved off the lustrous mane of hair, indicating that White women too understood the significance of long, kink-free hair.

As the lighter-skinned, straighter-haired slaves—men and women—continued to curry favor with the Whites in power, a skin-shade, hair-texture hierarchy developed within the social structure of the slave community. There were the light-skinned house slaves and the dark-skinned field slaves. The light-skinned slaves were said to have "good hair," and the dark-skinned slaves to have "bad hair." Good hair was thought of as long and lacking in kink, tight curls, and frizz. And the straighter the better. Bad hair was the antithesis, namely African hair in its purest form. White slave masters reinforced the "good-hair," light-skin power structure in two ways. By selecting the lighter-skinned, straighter-haired slaves for the best positions within his household, he showed they were more desirable. At slave auctions he would pay almost five times more for a house slave than for a field slave, showing they were also more valuable (a field hand could be bought for sixteen hundred dollars, while the going rate for a "fancy girl" was five thousand dollars). Black people themselves internalized the concept and within their own ranks propagated the notion that darker-skinned Blacks with kinkier hair were less attractive, less intelligent, and worth less than their lighterhued brothers and sisters. "We despise, we almost hate ourselves, and all that favors us," lamented one William J. Wilson in an article written in 1853 in *Frederick Douglass' Paper*. "Well may we scoff at black skins and woolly heads, since every model set before us for admiration, has a pallid face and flaxen head." By 1850 in the South, free mulattoes outnumbered slave mulattoes by two to one.

By the middle of the nineteenth century, a relatively small population of free Black Americans—clustered in urban centers in the North—were engaging in debates over the effects of light-skin, "good-hair" politics on Black identity. Already the practice of hair straightening was being questioned as the only option for mainstream society's acceptance. Martin H. Freeman voiced his doubts in the *Anglo-African* magazine:

> The child is taught directly or indirectly that he or she is pretty, just in proportion as the features approximate the Anglo-Saxon standard. Hence flat noses must be pinched up. Kinky hair must be subjected to a straightening process—oiled, and pulled, twisted up, tied down, sleeked over and pressed under, or cut off so short that it can't curl, sometimes the natural hair is shaved off and its place supplied by a straight wig. . . . Now all this is very foolish, perhaps wicked, but under the circumstances it is very natural.

Ironically, keeping the hair straight and in a close approximation of the mainstream styles of the day did very little to gain the acceptance or respect of White Americans. In fact, it often had the opposite effect. The free Black populations sprinkled about in cities like Boston and Philadelphia were wont to wear the same fashions and hairstyles as their White contemporaries only to find themselves ridiculed and satirized in the press, in the theaters, and on the streets. Blacks were actually accused of being pretentious in their adherence to White fashion standards. The culmination of this White derision was in the introduction of the minstrel show in the 1830s. White actors made up in blackface criticized and poked fun at the clothing, hairstyles, and physical behavior of well-dressed Black men and women—contemptuously termed *dandies*. Invented blackface characters like Zip Coon and Jim Crow became universal symbols of Black buffoonery across the country.

At the same time, those free Blacks with extremely light skin and straight hair, known as the "mulatto elite," still enjoyed a sense of freedom and riches unknown by Blacks with darker skin. Historian Joel Williamson writes that these "affluent" and "cultivated" Blacks "enjoyed a status markedly elevated above numbers of the free black mass." To maintain their precarious privilege, they were adept at segregating themselves in tight-knit communities. From New York to Louisiana, this Black elite protected its position in society by marrying only other Blacks with similar light coloring and straight hair, living in certain neighborhoods, and associating professionally and socially with similarly hued people. As far back as 1790, organizations were founded—like the Brown Fellowship Society in Charleston, South Carolina—whose criteria for entry were at least partially based on physical characteristics. A business networking group for Negro men, the Brown Fellowship was created by a group of free Black men, but membership was restricted to light-skinned Blacks. In response, those darker-hued men snubbed by the group formed the Society of Free Dark Men. By the time slavery was officially abolished in 1865, "good" hair and light skin had become the official keys to membership in the Negro elite.

Free at Last

Emancipation meant many things to the Black slaves of North America. With the promises of restitution and the opportunities offered through Reconstruction, the average Black person seemed to have the world at his or her feet. Of course this proved to be very far from the truth. Many Blacks actually felt they fared better under slavery than in the first years of freedom. "Most all the slaves had [a] place to live, clothes to wear, and plenty to eats [sic], and that is more than we has now," former slave Calvin Moye told a WPA interviewer. Sharecropping and menial labor were often the only options for the Black population in the rural South. Black people who were able to prosper still had to tread lightly around Whites so as not to provoke their jealousy or anger. And of course nobody wanted to attract the attention of the Ku Klux Klan. It was considered best for Blacks, especially men, to keep a low profile. Anything that a Black person had or did in excess was subject to the White majority's intense scrutiny. This was even true with regard to hair. In post–Civil War society, it was the fashion for White men to wear longer hair and beards, but when Black men allowed their hair to grow and stopped shaving off their facial hair (think Frederick Douglass), they were considered uppity and wild. On the other hand, Black women who attempted to style their hair in the long, prim, and proper styles of their White counterparts were considered well-adjusted by White society.

While White Americans took their time adapting to all Black people being "free," those tawny-hued Blacks who had been free for generations scrambled to solidify their position as an elite group. They immediately defined themselves as "bona fide" free Blacks, whereas the newly manumitted were termed "sot free." Needless to say, the "bona fides" did not mix with the "sot frees" and continued to establish schools, social organizations, and business networks where light skin and "good" hair were routinely the first criteria for entry. Even houses of worship were divided. Anecdotal evidence suggests that at this time "bona fide" churches sprang up where congregants had to pass a series of tests for membership. In some churches a fine-toothed comb was hung from the front door. All persons wanting to join the church had to be able to pass the comb smoothly through their hair. If their hair was too kinky, membership was denied. This was known as the comb test. There was also the brown-bag test, by which the skin was measured for lightness against a paper bag. During this time, historically Black colleges and universities like Howard (established in 1867), Hampton (1868), and Spelman (1881) were founded to educate the Black elite, but there too, judging from photographs of the early graduates, it seems as if one of the unspoken requirements for admission was a skin tone or hair texture that showcased a Caucasian ancestor.

The motivation for this intraracial discrimination stemmed from an unfortunately painful truth. White society, to some extent, was more accepting of lighter-skinned Blacks. It didn't help, however, that Black people, both light- and dark-skinned, helped perpetuate this truth by maintaining the straight-hair, light-skin hierarchy within their own ranks. Jobs, marriage partners, even education were typically predicated on the texture of the hair and the shade of the skin. Therefore, life after slavery for many Blacks meant a continued obsession with straightening the hair and lightening the skin. Now free to devote more time to their hair, Black men and women eagerly lavished attention on their locs and sought out the few commercial products now being manufactured exclusively for Black hair. Most Black people were desperate, in this time of potential prosperity, just to fit in with the crowd and make a decent life for themselves, firmly believing that a superficial cosmetic change could make a startling difference in the quality of their lives.

Advertisers—both White and Black—took advantage of the idea to sell hair straighteners and skin lighteners that promised not just to enhance one's beauty but to improve one's station in life. "You owe it to yourself, as well as to others who are interested in you, to make yourself as attractive as possible. Attractiveness will contribute much to your success—both socially and commercially," read a late-nineteenth-century advertisement for Curl-I-Cure hair preparations. In her book *Hair Raising*, Noliwe M. Rooks, a hair historian and visiting professor of African-American Studies at Princeton University, writes that in the late nineteenth century "advertisements for skin lighteners and hair straighteners marketed by White companies suggest to Blacks that only through changing physical features will persons of African descent be afforded class mobility within African-American communities and social acceptance by the dominant culture." The products being sold, like arsenic wafers for lightening the skin and lye for straightening the hair, were often dangerous chemical concoctions that not only failed to perform miracles but could prove deadly.

In the rural South, where an estimated 90 percent of the Black population continued to dwell after the Civil War, hair traditions continued as they had in slavery. Since many Blacks were still slaves to the land—employed as sharecroppers—a laborious, unhealthy antebellum lifestyle prevailed. The concept of personal time was still largely unknown. Women kept their braided hairstyles covered with a head rag, only to feel the light of day on Sundays and special occasions. Meanwhile in the northern cities, the Black men and women who had more access to professional hair salons and the few hair-care products on the market began to incorporate hairstyling into their daily routine. It was still a chore, but for the first time since the journey from Africa, Black hair could be celebrated outside the bonds of slavery.

A Helping of Good Old-Fashioned Black Hair Superstitions

1. Always burn the hair in your brush or someone could use it to put a hex on you.
2. Never comb, brush, or cut your hair outside because if a bird comes and collects a stray loc for its nest, you will:
   - Feel it pecking at your head
   - Get headaches
   - Lose your mind
   - Suffer the same fate as the bird's babies
3. Always wear your hair covered when menstruating.
4. If you allow more than one person to work on your hair at a time:
   - Your hair will fall out
   - The youngest worker/helper will die
5. Don't let a pregnant woman do your hair or you'll become pregnant too.
6. After someone finishes working on your hair, it's bad luck to say thank you. Instead, say "More hair."
7. Never cut a boy child's hair before age one or:
   - It won't grow
   - It will be kinky and nappy
8. After you cut your hair, if you place a loc in the Bible it will grow back faster.
9. It's bad luck for a woman to cut a man's hair, especially if she's menstruating.
10. If you want your hair to grow back, only cut it when there is a full moon.
11. If you get gray hair when you're young, it means you were a good baby.

2

No Excuse for Nappy:
1900–1964

In 1901 Sarah McWilliams, 34, was a widowed single mother with no formal education supporting a daughter in college on the income she made washing other people's clothes. Nine years later the *Guinness Book of World Records* hailed this very same woman as the first self-made female American millionaire. With inspiration gleaned from a fanciful dream, McWilliams, better known to the world as Madam C. J. Walker, came to symbolize all that Black hair stood for in the first half of the twentieth century. An avenue to success and respectability, Black nationalism and expression, controversy and heated debate, Black hair unleashed its power on an unsuspecting world.

The New Negro: 1900–1920

1900. It was a new year. A new century. And there was a New Negro.

Blacks in America had survived enslavement, a Civil War, and an emancipation that left them economically and politically at a crippling dis-advantage compared with Whites. Yet the twentieth century was the first time that Blacks were collectively a free people, able to exercise more than minimal control over their lives and destinies, albeit in a racist society. It was a time of promise and progress as well as one of hard work and the re-configuring of many ideas, norms, and ideologies. Blacks—no longer dis-tinguished as free or slave—began the century by shaping their collective identity. And the politics of appearance was to play a pivotal role.

To gain access to the American dream, one of the first things Blacks had to do was make White people more comfortable with their very pres-ence. It was not only Blacks who had been scarred by the racist stereo-types of the "savage Negro." Many Whites were frightened of Black people, and countless others exploited these fears to maintain the biased status quo. For White Americans, education and training made little differ-ence if a person looked too "African." Kinky hair, wide noses, and full lips translated to "ignorant," "uncivilized," and "infantile." "Taking on as many Eurocentric attributes as possible was a goal for the well-dressed person of color, man or woman," explains style expert Lloyd Boston, author of *Men of Color.* "The accepted image of the day was a well groomed White man [or woman]." So Blacks did what they could to emulate European standards of beauty, dress, and behavior.

"[Their] look was a calling card to make people feel comfortable and unthreatened," says Boston. The Negro elite and growing middle class had to fight hard to make impressions on the dominant society that would counter the negative, racist stereotypes that were imbedded in the main-stream collective consciousness. Besides mimicking the fashions of main-stream White society, Black men and women used various techniques to copy their hairstyles as well. "When it came to hair for African-Americans," says image consultant Harriette Cole, the goal was "to have hairstyles that were straight and then curled—organized, with every strand in place. That was something that was born out of a European aesthetic. So Blacks, par-ticularly middle-class [Black] people [who] were working and interacting with Whites, bought into that aesthetic and tried to become 'American' visually."

Some Black Americans with extremely light skin and straight, kink-free hair chose to break through the barriers that a racist society had con-structed by simply passing themselves off as White. Because of the wide-

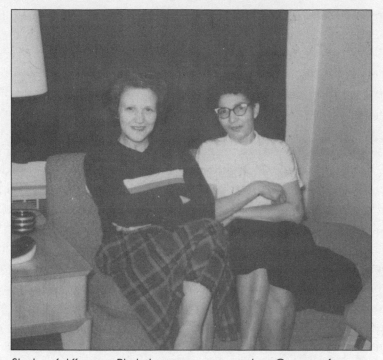

Shades of difference: Black skin comes in many colors. Courtesy of Florence Price.

spread miscegenation that had occurred during slavery, there were many members of the African-American community of the early 1900s who, for all intents and purposes, looked White. This phenomenon, called "passing," is defined as "the movement of a person who is legally or socially designated Black into a White racial category or White social identity." It has been estimated that in any given year, between ten thousand and thirty thousand Blacks chose this way of life. Yet many historians and social commentators note that it is not possible to know how many people actually passed. Nella Larsen's *Passing,* a classic novel of the Harlem Renaissance, is the story of two women, Clare and Irene. Clare has chosen to "become" White, while Irene passes occasionally. With Clare's blond hair and both women's pale skin, they are able to move with no problem across the boundaries separating Black and White society.

For those Blacks who chose not to pass, or who could not because of their telltale features, assimilation to a White aesthetic became the next best option. Black people fought the negative depictions put forth by the mainstream culture in many ways and most significantly through the construction of an alternative, oppositional appearance. This newly created image was termed the *New Negro*. Both an aspiration and an ideal, this image of the New Negro was a hybrid of retaliation and pride—retaliation against the negative images and caricatures put forth by White society about Blacks; pride in the achievements and respectability that many members of the race were attaining, despite tremendous odds. According to hair historian Noliwe Rooks, this image was "constructed to function as a model that others should emulate in attempting to better their condition within the larger American society." The New Negro, writes Rooks, was exemplified by the elite professional class who were "committed to defining identities for an African-American populace." Ideally, through the attainment of these qualities, Black people would be accepted into those areas of society, both economic and political, to which racist Whites had denied them access. In many ways, then, this concept of the New Negro became a survival tactic, a maneuver to infiltrate forbidden territory while simultaneously redefining an image. The hair, having been subjected for nearly three hundred years to both creative and at times damaging experiments in the quest for straightness and "manageability," was a key element in the construction of this New Negro image.

While men were often the ones being hailed as the leaders of the race, it was the New Negro woman who became, in many ways, its symbol. In cultures throughout the world, women, who are the least enfranchised in a society, are commonly used to represent the norms and values of the group. Therefore Black Womanhood, a construct so diminished by the rapes and other abuses of slavery, was rebuilt and revered as a symbol of the Civilized Negro. In 1900 educator and businessman Booker T. Washington edited a volume entitled *A New Negro for a New Century*, in which he stated that "the African-American woman can prove to the world that Negro Womanhood when properly treated and educated will burst forth into gems of pure brilliancy unsurpassed by any other race." What did this Face for the Race have to look like? In many ways, and not surprisingly since the light-skinned Black elite heavily influenced these ideas, the idealized Black woman had many Eurocentric features, including hairstyles. According to A'Lelia Bundles, biographer and great-great-granddaughter of Madam C. J. Walker, the ideal woman of the late nineteenth and early twentieth century had a "great mass of hair, which she swept to the top of her head." For those women of any race that were unable to attain this look naturally, there was a thriving wig and hairpiece industry to assist them. "The dressing of one's hair should be a matter of deep concern," stated the popular beauty guide *A Complete Course in Hair Straightening and Beauty Culture.* "To no other race is this more important than the Negro woman."

While Black women's physical appearance symbolically represented more for the race, Black men too dedicated significant amounts of time to hair-care regimens. For the first two decades of the twentieth century, Black men sought to slicken, straighten, and otherwise style their hair through the use of tonics and pomades. A 1911 advertisement in the Black newspaper *The Age* asks, "Have you had your hair straightened yet? Up and around 135th and Lenox Avenue colored men can be seen in large numbers who are wont to take off their hats repeatedly . . . and stroke their glossy hair with their hand in an affectionate manner." While there were some haircuts that did not require such an arsenal of products, men looking to style their hair usually found it necessary first to alter the texture from its original state. "Cold soap" waves were a popular method for achieving the pronounced parts and sleek looks of the time. These waves were achieved by washing the hair, not rinsing out all the soap, and wearing do-rags (cloth rags tied over the head to produce pressurized wave patterns). Another popular straightening technique for men was to comb or brush large quantities of hair grease and water through the hair at night and then cover it in a do-rag as they slept.

No Excuse for Nappy

In this new era, led by a "bootstrap mentality" in which Black people collectively worked toward carving a place for themselves in the land that had enslaved them one generation earlier, there was no excuse for "nappy," or unstraightened, hair. Writer Azalia Hackley noted in the early 1900s that while "kinky hair is an honorable legacy from Africa," it was nonetheless a trait she hoped "constant care" would help make to go away. Looking respectable was not just an individual pursuit. At this time in history more so than any other, Blacks were being judged as a monolithic group and the actions or appearance of one was seen as a reflection of the whole.

Advertisements for hair treatments and cosmetics reflected this we're-all-in-it-together mentality. For example, an ad in the Black newspaper *The Oklahoma Eagle* declared, "Amazing Progress of Colored Race—Improved Appearance Responsible. Look your best . . . you owe it to your race." The appearance, including the hair, was the means to a socioeconomic end. "African-American people who felt that they were lucky to get any kind of professional job understood and believed that to be a cookie cutter as best they could of White America would at least present an opportunity," explains Harriette Cole.

By the early 1900s, straight hair had become the preferred look to signal middle-class status. There was an overwhelmingly large number of lighter-skinned Blacks who made up the upper class and the so-called Negro elite. Just as in the days of slavery, the hierarchy in social and class status could often be ascertained by skin tone and hair texture. "Even among intelligent Negroes there has come into being the fallacious belief that black Negroes are less able to achieve success," wrote American anthropologist Melville J. Herskovits in a 1925 essay, "The Negro's Americanism." "Naturally such a condition has led to jealousy and suspicion on the part of darker Negroes, chafing at their bonds and resentful of the patronizing attitude of those of lighter color." Light-skinned Blacks represented the majority of the two thousand plus African-American college graduates, twenty-one thousand schoolteachers, and thirty-five thousand ministers living in America by 1900.

The Birth of the Black Hair-Care Boom

Promised forty acres and a mule at Emancipation, most African-Americans entered the twentieth century with considerably less. As the century progressed, the creation of a Black consumer market, an obvious outgrowth of a rising middle class, was to have a major impact on the role of Black hair and the significance attached to it. With disposable income, more Blacks had the means to purchase cosmetics, namely bleaching creams and hair-straightening products. With the attainment and use of these goods, they were able to work toward achieving the respectable look of the New Negro.

As the quest for social and economic mobility continued, hair became a

means by which many would build their fortunes, or at the very least ensure that there would be food on the table every night. The turn of the
century saw the entrance of numerous Black-owned companies (including
the Overton Hygienic Manufacturing Company and Winona Hair Empo-
rium) into a field previously dominated by White firms (such as Curl-
I-Cure and Kinkilla). Yet it is the stories of two hair-care capitalists, Annie
Turnbo Malone and Madam C. J. Walker, that best illustrate the way Black
hair was used to make money while simultaneously helping to build up the
race. The story of these two women also illuminates a theme that will be
seen throughout the modern history of Black hair in America—the contra-
dictions that seem to lie at the core of creating an industry that is pro-Black
while pushing an agenda of altering or "improving" on Black features by
making them appear "whiter."

Annie Minerva Turnbo Malone was born on a farm in Metropolis, Illinois,
in 1869, the tenth of eleven children. Orphaned at an early age, she was
raised by an older sister in Peoria, Illinois. In the late 1890s Malone, who
was said to have a background in chemistry, began to concoct recipes for
products that would solve the hair problems, such as baldness and breakage, that many Black women of the time faced as a result of a high-stress
lifestyle, a nutritionally deficient diet, and inadequate hygiene. As a young
woman, Malone was dissatisfied with the hair-care remedies and styling
techniques that were available. She wanted to find a product that would
make hair more "manageable" at a time when getting the hair into new
styles each day posed a challenge, considering that even running water was
a luxury for many Blacks. This was before the permanent chemical straightener, a good jar of grease, the hot comb, or the Afro pick were readily available, and getting a comb through kinky curls was not always a simple thing
to do. By 1900 Malone had developed a product that she claimed would
make hair grow. Calling it Wonderful Hair Grower, she began selling her
new "miracle cure" door-to-door in the town of Lovejoy, Illinois. Its immediate success marked the beginning of Malone's entrance into the hair-
care industry, and she soon expanded her product line.

In 1902 thirty-three-year-old Malone moved her base of operations to
Saint Louis, where the new business flourished. She named the company
Poro, which is a Mende (West African) word meaning "devotional society."

(It is interesting that, at a time when many Blacks were looking to cast off connections to Africa, Malone would embrace a Mende word for her company's title.) After a nine-month tour of the South to expand her market, she adopted a sales strategy that was being used throughout the nation by a number of female entrepreneurs. Malone would train and certify an agent in how to use her products and methods for hair care. These women would then earn money by selling the hair treatments door-to-door and retaining a percentage of the profits. Any person who had completed the Poro training course could also open an official Poro salon. To increase their profits, experienced agents, who would receive a commission on all new recruits, signed up new women to take the Poro course. In a short time Poro products were being sold across the country and eventually throughout the Caribbean and Latin America. Malone's business and marketing approach was so successful that in 1906 she trademarked the name Poro in order to ward off, in her own words, "fradulent imitators."

The Poro Company was successful for reasons beyond making a profit. Malone was one of the first successful African-American women who sought to increase her income while simultaneously giving other Black women a viable way to make money. She offered incentives, including diamond rings and gold plaques, to top-selling agents and instilled a sense of pride into those who completed the training process. Diplomas hung on the walls of many graduates of the Malone agent training. She supported and created commercial opportunities and networks in women's clubs, churches, and schools, and she founded an orphanage. In 1924 she gave a twenty-five-thousand-dollar donation to the Saint Louis Colored YMCA. Malone's greatest contribution, however, was the 1917 erection of Poro College in Saint Louis, an immense multimillion-dollar complex that housed her manufacturing plant, sales operations, and the first U.S. school for training African-American hairstylists and agents, as well as a gymnasium, chapel, and a space for theater, concerts, and lectures. Poro College doubled as company headquarters and a community center for the Black residents of Saint Louis.

Malone's success did not go unnoticed. Many people, Black and White, tried to follow in her entrepreneurial footsteps. One woman in particular was taking copious notes. She was known as Madam C. J. Walker.

Madam C. J. Walker was born Sarah Breedlove on a cotton plantation near Delta, Louisiana, in 1867. Orphaned at the age of seven, married at fourteen, and a widow by twenty, Breedlove and her daughter, Lelia, existed on her meager earnings as a laundress in Saint Louis, Missouri. Like many Black women at the time, Breedlove (who now went by the name McWilliams after her deceased husband, Moses McWilliams) suffered from hair that was short and patchy, revealing her scalp in several places. She believed that if she could improve her appearance, she could build her self-confidence and consequently improve her station in life. She was inspired by the impressive appearance of Margaret Murray Washington, wife of Booker T. Washington, whom she had seen address the Saint Louis branch of the National Association of Colored Women in 1904. McWilliams decided that a major step toward improving her appearance would be finding a way to fix

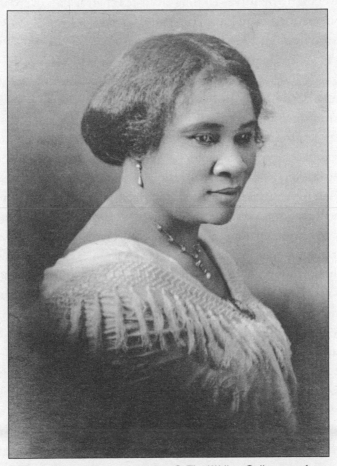

Madam C. J. Walker, circa 1914. © The Walker Collection of A'Lelia Bundles.

her damaged, sparse hair. She began using a number of the products on the market that claimed to grow hair, including some Poro products, and for a short time McWilliams even became a Poro agent, selling Poro's Wonderful Hair Grower.

After a year of unsuccessful attempts to make her hair long and full, McWilliams was still looking for a remedy for her damaged tresses and was as determined as ever to leave the life of a laundress behind. One night in 1905 she had a dream. "God answered my prayer," she was to explain to a reporter. "For one night I had a dream, and in that dream a big Black man appeared to me and told me what to mix up for my hair. Some of the remedy was grown in Africa, but I sent for it, mixed it, put it on my scalp and in a few weeks my hair was coming in faster than it had ever fallen out." After testing the mixture on friends with satisfactory results, McWilliams decided to go into business for herself. Fearful that the Saint Louis market was oversaturated Poro territory, she looked for a new place to start and chose to move to Denver, where her older brother lived. Once there, she immediately began door-to-door sales. Now calling herself Madam C. J. Walker after marrying her third husband, adman Charles J. Walker, she advertised the products in Black newspapers and began a mail-order business. She made the hair preparations in her kitchen from that recipe that came to her through divine intervention. Traveling around the South and Midwest, talking about and demonstrating her products and training agents, Walker and her company prospered. In 1908 she and daughter, Lelia, moved the company headquarters to Pittsburgh and opened the Lelia College, a beauty parlor and training school for Walker agents, dubbed "hair culturists." Within a few years, Lelia Colleges had opened in Indianapolis and New York. In 1910 Walker, now divorced, moved the company headquarters to Indianapolis and enlarged her product line to include Hair Grower (her top seller), Glossine (a pomade), Vegetable Shampoo, Tetter Salve (an antidandruff treatment), and Temple Grower.

Walker sealed her place in Black hair history with the introduction of the Walker system, the "shampoo-press-and-curl" method of straightening hair that was to become the foundation of the Black beautician industry. The central component of the system was a kit sold to those men and women who had passed the Walker training course. Among other items, the kit included a hot comb. A hot comb is a metal comb that is heated on a range top or burner and then pulled through the hair to straighten it temporarily. Walker is often erroneously credited with inventing the comb, when in fact it was created by the French in the nineteenth century, intended for the ladies of Paris during a time of revived interest in the poker-straight Egyptian hairstyles of the past. Hot combs had been available for retail sale in the United States since the 1880s, when catalogs for companies like Bloomingdales and Sears featured the item. Walker's company, which acquired the combs from different suppliers across the country, was largely responsible for introducing the comb to Black women. Until Walker Manufacturing began promoting the comb, Black women had been straightening their hair with old-time slavery methods as well as with instruments called "pullers," a tool championed by Annie Turnbo Malone. Walker cautioned against the use of these round tongs and warned in her training literature that pullers would "pull and flatten out [the hair] which closes the glands which prevents nourishment and will finally cause it to become very thin."

With the success of the Walker system and the subsequent growth of Walker Manufacturing, Madam C. J. Walker moved into the ranks of the Negro elite. At a time when the average uneducated Black woman made less than ten dollars a week, Walker built herself a $250,000 thirty-four-room mansion on the Hudson River, owned four automobiles, including an electric coupé, and two other homes. A frequent donor to various charities, including the National Association for the Advancement of Colored People (NAACP), Walker also erected a community center for the Black residents of Indianapolis.

It is important to note that, while mavericks in many ways, neither Malone, Walker, nor the numerous other successful Black hair-care entrepreneurs challenged the prevailing notions of beauty that existed at the time. Instead they sought to create safe, affordable products that would give all classes of Black women the means of achieving this straight-haired ideal. Walker emphasized to her agents that they should pamper their clients so they felt beautiful both inside and out. "To be beautiful," Walker stressed, "does not refer alone to the arrangement of the hair, the perfection of the complexion or to the beauty of the form. . . . To be beautiful, one must combine these qualities with a beautiful mind and soul." This was a new concept for Black Americans, who had been routinely denied the luxury of beauty rituals.

Many critics fault Walker for making her fortune by telling Black women that they needed to straighten their hair. This criticism is only reasonable if the situation is taken out of historical context. Walker and Malone were not responsible for creating the idea that Black hair had to be straight to look presentable. Many factors went into the development of the idea that kinky hair was unacceptable. Malone and Walker were two women who were not of mixed heritage, did not have naturally straight or wavy hair, and like many other women were faced with ineffective or harmful products with which to care for their hair. They both understood that a woman, especially a darker-skinned woman with short hair that was dry and brittle and showed bald spots, had a harder time securing a job, finding a husband, or even walking down the street with pride. They were looking not only to make money but also to provide the women of their race with the means to change their appearance and consequently their lot in life. Both women recognized the importance of a neat, handsome hairdo for social acceptability. "I make hair grow," Walker told a reporter for the *Indianapolis Recorder*. "I want the great masses of my people to take a greater pride in their appearance and to give their hair proper attention." However, Walker maintained throughout her lifetime that she was not interested in whether or not people straightened their hair. "Her advertisements never even used the word 'straight.' [She wasn't] recommending that everybody go buy a [hot] comb," explains A'Lelia Bundles. Walker's ultimate goal, aside from making sales, was to make Black women feel good about how they looked.

A Contested Ideal

While precious few examples of Black style were present in the mainstream media, the Black press, beauty pageants, and local fashion shows were instrumental in keeping people up-to-date on the latest looks. *Half Century Magazine*, a leading African-American magazine of the first quarter of the twentieth century, never had a cover model with unstraightened hair, although a range of skin tones were displayed. Beauty contests and pageants at this time, including those that stressed they were celebrating all types of racial beauty, featured contestants only with straight hair. Cornrows, plaits, and other styles that were common in the 1800s were now found only on older rural women in the South. As large groups of Blacks moved to northern cities, they made sure that their hair was done in the latest straight styles so as not to look "countrified" in their new urban homes. As A'Lelia Bundles explains, "If you are a rural person becoming an urban person then you [want to] look less like a person from the country, less like an uneducated person."

The *practice* of straightening the hair, however, was a highly contested issue within the Black community. Everyone had an opinion, including members of the Black elite, politicians, ministers, and intellectuals. The debate was waged in church services, in the media, on back porches, and in kitchens across the country. Prominent Black women's groups went so far as to form Anti-Hair-Wrapping Clubs, organizations dedicated to the eradication of the practice of straightening the hair by wrapping a heated piece of flannel on an oiled head. Although many Black leaders were in favor of the increased attention to grooming and appearance in the fight for social acceptance, many denounced hair straightening as a pitiful attempt to emulate Whites and equated hair straightening with self-hatred and shame. Nannie Helen Burroughs, founder of the National Training School for Girls and Women, wrote in a 1904 article titled "Not Color But Character" that "What every woman who . . . straightens out needs, is not her appearance changed but her mind changed. . . . If Negro women would use half of the time they spend on trying to get White, to get better, the race would move forward."

Booker T. Washington directed his anger not at the Blacks who straightened but at the manufacturers that made straightening products, on the grounds that they promoted a White standard of beauty. Washington initially went so far as to ban beauty "culturists" from working as instructors at his famed Tuskegee Institute, a school created for the purpose of teaching various trades to African-Americans. Owners of hair-care product firms were also for a time denied membership in Washington's National Negro Business League (NNBL), an organization dedicated to the task of promoting Black commerce, even though hairdressing for both men and women proved to be one of the most profitable postslavery Black-owned enterprises. In 1912 an indignant Madam Walker demanded that she be heard and recognized at the NNBL's annual convention. "Surely you are not going to shut the door in my face," she exclaimed to Washington after three days of trying to get the attention of the convention participants. Walker went on to tell the audience that she "came from the cotton fields of the South" and that she knew "how to grow hair as well as I know how to grow cotton. I have built my own factory on my own ground." But while Walker captured the attention of the convention attendees, her speech did not immediately change Washington's general feeling that the profession did not qualify as a legitimate means of pulling oneself up by one's bootstraps. Critics of Washington note that sexism may have influenced his decision to single out and denounce the only industry that was dominated by women.

Meanwhile, as nationalist organizations, such as W. E. B. DuBois's Pan-African movement, developed a larger following into the 1920s, the politics of appearance, namely skin bleaching and hair straightening, became more contentious among Blacks, particularly in the North. In her examination of America's beauty culture, *Hope in a Jar*, Kathy Peiss writes that "Emphasizing race pride, educators considered [hair straightening and skin bleaching] a degrading bid to deny African heritage and to look like White people. Ministers railed against those who practiced and profited from these unnatural and ungodly habits." Black nationalist Marcus Garvey, leader of the United Negro Improvement Association (UNIA), made the reclamation of an African-based aesthetic a central tenet of his political platform. "Don't remove the kinks from your hair!" he once proclaimed in a speech. "Remove them from your brain!" The pages of Black newspapers during this time were full of letters and editorials on the hair straightening controversy. The Black news journal *Crusader* weighed in by featuring women wearing traditional African hair arrangements on its covers.

There was, however, a definite strain of contradiction running throughout this ongoing public debate over hair straightening. For instance, W. E. B. DuBois, who criticized the Black masses for "always looking at oneself through the ideas of others," had naturally wavy hair, as did the overwhelming majority of those who comprised the "talented tenth," those Black thinkers and artists who DuBois felt would be the leaders of the race. The wives of many of the ministers who shouted from their pulpits that straightening the hair was the work of the devil were heavy consumers of straightening potions and beauty shop services. Marcus Garvey, who fiercely denounced straight hair, owned and operated a newspaper, *Negro World*, that devoted approximately two-thirds of its advertising to hair products, including straighteners. And Garvey's *Negro World* was not the only Black newspaper that filled its pages with text that condemned straightening yet carried advertising for straightening products. The NAACP's *Crisis* magazine was but one example of the many publications chock-full of advertisements for "image enhancers."

At the same time, Black civic leaders were not the only group angered by the latest trends in hair care. As the proliferation of hair-care products and hot combs spread across the country, many older rural Southern women were also displeased. In a WPA interview, former slave Jane Michens Toombs remarked that "if a [Negro] wanted to get the kinks out of their hair they combed it with the cards. Now they put all kinds of grease on it, an' buy straightenin' combs. . . . Old fashion cards'll straighten hair just as well as all this high smellin stuff they sell now." As the Black migration to the North continued in the 1920s, many of those still living in the South saw the new straightened, high-glossed styles as an indication of trying to look "citified." Their argument against these products was not a pronationalist stance but one based on an aversion to urbanization.

Arguments about hair straightening and the success of manufacturing products for this purpose in the early twentieth century must also take into consideration the overall growth of the American cosmetic industry. Getting "made up," including both cosmetics and hairstyling, was a common practice at this time for American women in all walks of life, regardless of region or race. What had once been the practice only of "loose," immoral women was now hardly noticed. In straightening their hair and buying into the consumer culture, Black women, it could be said, were merely becoming more "modern." A 1920 editorial in *Half Century Magazine* upheld this idea. "Thousands of White women have their hair straightened because it is quite impossible to 'do up' any but the straightest of hair in some of the most approved styles. Colored women have their hair straightened for the same reason. . . . Most White women feel that they would rather be dead than out of style and in that respect their darker sisters do not differ from them one iota." Consequently, the debate over straightening could be said to be less about the emulation of Whites than about the embracing of modernity.

Anthropologists Shane and Graham White offer yet another interpretation of the straightening ritual. "Straightening the hair may be seen not as a sign of a defective Black consciousness but as an integral part of a time-honored creative process," they assert in *Stylin'*. Hair has historically been a medium of adornment for people of African descent, so straightening could be considered just one of a long list of styling options. As Harriette

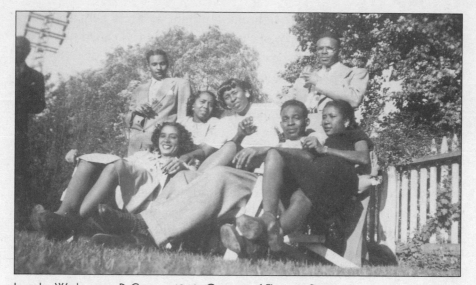

In style: Washington, D.C., circa 1940. Courtesy of Florence Price.

Cole notes, "It wasn't just about looking like White folks. [Blacks] always put a creative spin on it." The styles that Black women and men wore after straightening their hair rarely mirrored the looks of their White counterparts. This was particularly true with men. Their straightened hair, often with dyed reddish hues and slicked-back sides, was visually nothing like the styles worn by White men or any other race. In straightening their hair, Black men had created a look that was wholly unique—it was neither naturally textured nor "White" hair. Even the marcelled wave style, first popularized by White women, looked altogether distinct when adopted by African-American women. Yet these styles, these latest contributions to the "time-honored creative process" of Black hairstyling, required straightening. In *Half Century Magazine*, in an article entitled "The Arrangement of the Coiffure," beauty editor Evelyn Northington counsels readers that "Unless [the] hair be of very good quality, it is almost impossible to arrange it artistically without the use of the straightening comb."

The matter of straightened versus natural hair may have been an ideological or political issue for Black civic and political leaders and a symbol of success and opportunity for the elite, but for many average Black folks, hair was a key factor in issues of self-esteem. Straight hair was slick, modern, and attractive. The beauty ideal that existed at the time overwhelmingly favored a light-skinned, straight-haired aesthetic for both men and women. Advertising throughout the first half of the century, as well as popular culture figures and images, did not offer an alternative Black beauty ideal. Many African-Americans were left with feelings of inadequacy and shame. As is the case throughout all levels of American society, although both men and women were evaluated by this standard it was traditionally women who internalized it, as women are most commonly evaluated on looks first and all other criteria second. In Wallace Thurman's 1929 novel *The Blacker the Berry*, the author gives a fictionalized account of the searing psychological effects on a young woman, Emma Lou, born into a "blue vein" (extremely fair-skinned) family "cursed" with the "crow-like" dark-skinned complexion of her father. Her only redemption is in her hair, "a thick, curly black mass . . . rich and easily controlled." Unable to command respect from others and to navigate successfully through the prejudices of her world, Emma Lou's lack of confidence stemmed from her perceived unattractiveness. An excerpt from Maya Angelou's autobiography *I Know Why the Caged Bird Sings* captures the internalized pain and anger that many Blacks experienced. Angelou writes of growing up in the 1930s: "Wouldn't they be surprised when one day I woke up out of my black ugly dream, and my real hair, which was long and blonde, would take the place of the kinky mass that mama wouldn't let me straighten? . . . Because I was really White and because a cruel fairy stepmother, who was understandably jealous of my beauty, had turned me into a too-big Negro girl, with nappy hair, broad feet and a space between her teeth that would hold a number-two pencil."

Straightening It Out: 1945–1964

Though debates over the meaning of it raged on, Black hair remained a near obsession for African-Americans. More than a cause of sociopolitical debate, hair had an effect on many different areas of life. A woman could not obtain work as a dancer at some nightclubs in Harlem if she did not have a certain hair texture. During World War II, the U.S. military—responding to intense demand by Black GIs stationed around the world—granted special permission to Murray's Cosmetic Company to obtain "vital and scarce materials" for the manufacturing of its popular Hair Pomade. After the bombing of Pearl Harbor, the United States stopped the importation of hair for attachments and wigs from China, a move that seriously reduced the hairstyle options for many African-American women. These few examples highlight the pervasiveness of the issue and how something so seemingly innocuous as a hairstyle could reverberate through unexpected levels of society.

The Black press contributed greatly to the prime position that hair enjoyed. Perusing any Black paper or journal of the time, one would find an exorbitant number of advertisements promoting hair-care products. In most of these publications, according to Noliwe Rooks, more than 50 percent of their advertising was for cosmetics and toiletries, including bleaches and straighteners. The money these newspapers made from selling this ad space proved invaluable in keeping the Black presses rolling.

Black men, as the Murray's Hair Pomade story illustrates, played a large role on the consumer side of the hair issue. For years African-American men had been paying a noticeable amount of attention to their hair. In *The Blacker the Berry*, Wallace Thurman creates the character of Braxton, a Harlem playboy who dedicates most of his time to polishing his appearance. Satirizing the excesses of some men's cosmetic rituals, Thurman describes how Braxton "had been preparing himself in his usual bedtime manner. His face had been cold-creamed, his hair greased and tightly covered by a silken stocking cap." Like their female counterparts, many Black men were looking to straighten their hair. These were, according to Lloyd Boston, "well-groomed men who shared the same belief that straight hair was more manageable, offered more styling possibilities, and was simply more attractive than their natural texture." For some of these men, the interest in straight hair was to look "hip" and in touch with the latest trends. For the first time since Blacks had been in America, African-American men, especially those living in urban centers such as New York and Chicago, were able to dedicate some time to the art of dressing themselves up. This included styling their hair. Others, however, knew the necessity of visual conformity when presenting themselves to the White world. Harriette Cole explains, "It was not that they were trying to be White, but they wanted to be professional."

The straightening methods of earlier decades for men—wave caps and cold curls—were losing popularity because they required such constant maintenance. In keeping with the explosion of the beauty product market, soon Black men had a permanent solution. It was called the congalene, or conk for short, and was a caustic solution of potatoes, eggs, and lye. One of the first commercially available conks was created by a company called KKK (Knocks Kinks Krazy) that was based in Los Angeles and owned by two Black entertainers named Peg Leg Bates and Mr. Roe. Lafayette Jones, former executive director of the American Health and Beauty Aids Institute (AHBAI), told *Shades of Beauty* magazine that "The name KKK was an in-joke, a way of diffusing something that struck terror into the hearts of Blacks." Few found the joke funny, so while the product, Konkalene, was groundbreaking in what it could do, it did not fly off the shelves. Another of the early conks was created by a Harlem barber known simply as Hart, and it soon became a preferred brand for musicians and entertainers.

Many Black men, to save money, took to making homemade conks instead of buying the ones available on the market. Mixing a recipe of two white potatoes, an egg, and Red Devil Lye, future Black nationalist Malcolm X and his friend Shorty gave the young Malcolm his first conk in the late 1940s. "My head caught fire. I gritted my teeth and tried to pull the sides of the kitchen table together. The comb felt as if it was raking my skin off. . . . My knees were trembling," he wrote in his autobiography. But in the end he deemed the result worth the pain. "I'd seen some pretty conks, but when it's the first time, on your *own* head, the transformation, after the lifetime of kinks, is staggering," he remembered. While Malcolm X's account is by far the most famous retelling of the extremes that men went through for the style, it is definitely not the only one. In their quest for straight hair, countless men subjected themselves to the scalding combination of ingredients. It was a style that took hold in the late twenties, peaked in the heyday of the zoot suit forties, and did not lose its popularity until well into the sixties. Cab Calloway, Nat King Cole, Little Richard, and countless other men in the public eye validated the look as one of style and hipness.

Black hair for men and women in the first six-plus decades of the twentieth century did not undergo many styling changes. For a short time around World War I the bald look was in vogue, popularized by African-American boxer Jack Johnson, and as previously noted some men were experimenting with "processes," or conked styles. Yet overwhelmingly the look was either a short cut or a slicked-back straightened style. Women's magazines, such as *Half Century*, dedicated pages to telling their readers how to best care for their hair. The instructions were elementary: brush your hair every night, wash it at least every two weeks, never straighten hair that is not clean and completely dry. These beauty columns were more interested in basic grooming techniques than actual styles. Hairpieces, called "switches," and wigs were available by mail order and in certain beauty shops to lengthen or shorten one's look, but what was most important was how straight, neat, and shiny the hair was. *How* you wore your hair was of much less consequence than how unnapped it was.

Basic styles for women were based on a croquinole curl (in which curlers called "croquinoles" are used to curl the hair tightly) that was combed into waves or a pageboy (in which longer hair is straightened and then curled under at the ends). Short hair was pressed and then put into tight curls that were combed out. The hairpiece industry had been a thriving one since the 1800s. At the turn of the century, when piling masses of hair on top of the head was in vogue, Black and White women bought switches. When the flapper look was popularized in the twenties, short cuts came into fashion. This was a welcome relief, according to *Half Century Magazine*, for the women who had "burned off and pulled out so much hair in the last few years." Some women, whose own hair had never grown to the lengths that past looks demanded, eagerly adopted the short cuts. Others, who had invested precious time and money into growing their hair long, bought switches and wigs to simulate the short flapper cut. Those women who did not want to sacrifice any hair to the scissors could buy attachable bangs (short fringes of hair that fall over the forehead). When the importing of hair attachments and wigs ground to a halt after Pearl Harbor, women remained in the shorter, sleeker styles worn by celebrities such as Lena Horne and Dorothy Dandridge. These short, tapered looks were to stay popular through the late 1940s, when there was resurgence of interest in attachments, now called "falsies." A 1947 *Ebony* article reported that more than four million Black women bought an average of two falsies a year made of raw hair from China, Italy, Czechoslovakia, Sweden, and Norway. The biggest market was the southeastern United States. However, costly wigs (some as high as twenty-seven dollars) were more popular in the Northeast.

In 1947, as the falsie market was growing, manufacturers were looking for a product that would permanently ensure that hair stayed as unnappy as possible. Straightened hair, especially for women, had its downside.

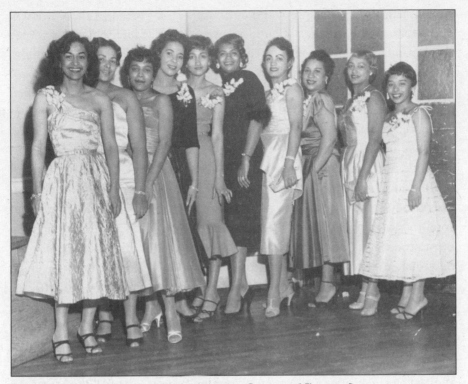

Stepping out: Philadelphia nightlife, early 1950s. Courtesy of Florence Price.

When straightened hair regained its kink, usually because of humidity, wet weather, or activities such as swimming or sweating, it was called "turning back." Former president of Planned Parenthood Faye Wattleton, in a *Harper's Bazaar* article from 1995, recounts the problem of traveling and maintaining straight hair in the days before chemical straighteners. "My mother came prepared with a small liquid-fuel burner that could be fired behind the closed doors of our room to heat the comb that would remove the natural curl of my 'nappy' hair," she says of the daily ritual before attending evening church meetings. "'Hold still!' my mother would command, as I dodged the searing straightening comb." A Philadelphia woman, Rochelle Nichols Solomon, remembers attending dances and how "when the lights came on at the end of the night—a night of nonstop dancing and sweating—people would scatter like rats." In response to the dilemmas of "turning back," the White-owned Lustrasilk company introduced its Lustrasilk Permanent in 1947, a product that purported to keep the hair straight longer than the regular press-and-curl method. It promised that "life will be different with Lustrasilk" and showed in its advertisements a "free" Black woman dancing, working, and playing tennis with perfectly straight, unfrizzy hair. Not to be outdone, Walker Manufacturing debuted its Satin Tress with great fanfare and an aggressive advertising campaign less than one year later. Ironically, both products required the use of a hot comb to straighten the hair. Furthermore, neither made the expected impression on consumers, but they paved the way for numerous imitators and, eventually, groundbreaking improvements. By the mid-1960s there were numerous products available, such as Johnson Products' top-selling Ultra Sheen Relaxer, for those looking to straighten their tresses chemically without combs or heat. While harsh lye bases and costly, time-consuming upkeep prevented these "perms" from being the perfect solution to a century-old dilemma, their creation nonetheless changed Black hair culture forever.

As the century rolled along, there were many changes in the African-American experience, yet one thing that did not dramatically alter was the attitude toward hair. The debates put forth by the nationalists of the 1920s had not produced significant changes. "Good" and "bad" hair were still a part of the African-American lexicon. A 1947 advertisement for Snow White Hair Beautifier warns men "Don't be 'Wire-Haired Willie,' the man nobody loves!" with a "before" photo of a man with hair standing on end and a surprised Sambo-like expression on his face and an "after" shot of a glossy, straight 'do and a big smile. Blacks still consciously sought to present White America with alternative images to the racist depictions of popular culture. Yet mainstream America was still pouring out cultural images such as Buckwheat, the ultra nappy-headed, poorly talking, dimwitted Black character in *The Little Rascals*. Images like Buckwheat were mere updates of the Sambos, Coons, and other minstrel show characters of the past.

Within the Black community, straight hair was not only the preferred look but a marker of one's position in society. Light skin and straight hair still represented wealth, education, and access to the upper echelons of society. Institutions of higher education were still common sites for intraracial discrimination. At Black colleges, whether or not there was an official or unofficial standard for skin color and hair texture, it was estimated that as early as 1916, 80 percent of students were light-skinned and of mixed heritage. Fraternities and sororities became another site for playing out color and hair elitism. The Alpha Kappa Alpha sorority and Kappa Alpha Psi fraternity acquired the reputation of being the light-skinned, "good"-hair groups. Black Greeks created "color-tax" parties in the twenties. At these parties, men would have to pay a tax determined by how dark their dates were. In a slight variation on this, Lawrence Otis Graham, author of *Our Kind of People*, tells of Black fraternity parties where attendees were let in based on a "ruler test." Only partygoers whose hair was as straight as a ruler would be admitted.

Although it was still politics as usual in many areas when it came to appearance, there was change on the horizon. Men such as Cassius Clay, the young, brash heavyweight fighter who soon renamed himself Muhammad Ali, were emerging as symbols of heroism and style for a new generation of African-Americans in the late 1950s. These men were Black entertainers who wore their hair in short, unstraightened styles. For some, such as Isaac Hayes, who traded his conk in for a baldie at this time, the shift away from straight hair was largely a cosmetic change. For others, however, it was emblematic of a slow resurgence in Black nationalist thought that once again deemed straight hair as equivalent to self-hatred.

Echoing the ideas of the nationalist movements of the 1920s, many groups, particularly the Nation of Islam, once again brought the politics of appearance to the forefront of Black America's social consciousness. The Nation said that Whites had taught Black Americans to hate themselves and therefore come to believe that they were inferior to Whites, by convincing them that Africa and all things African, including kinky hair, were bad. Malcolm X, who was now a leading figure in the Nation, had stopped straightening his own hair and come to see that day when he had burned his scalp to get his first conk as the "first really big step toward self-degradation: when I endured all of that pain, literally burning my flesh to have it look like a White man's hair. I had joined that multitude of Negro men and women in America who are [so] brainwashed into believing that the Black people are 'inferior' . . . that they will even violate and mutilate their God-created bodies to try to look 'pretty' by White standards." As he once said, "We hated our African characteristics. We hated our hair. We hated the shape of our nose, and the shape of our lips, the color of our skin. . . . This is how [Whites] imprisoned us. Not just bringing us over here and making us slaves. But the image that you created of our motherland and the image that you created of our people on that continent was a trap, was a prison, was a chain, was the worst form of slavery that has ever been invented. . . ." Malcolm X maintained through speeches and writings that Blacks who had been "colonized mentally" would not be able to break the chains of racism until they learned to love their appearance.

Teachings such as these were spreading throughout the cities of the North—and New York's Harlem neighborhood in particular—at the same time that the Civil Rights movement was mobilizing citizens in the South. The message of integration to White America was that "we are American people too." Integration leaders were not interested in presenting White America with an "Africanized" people, but the movement did instill a much needed sense of Black pride in the race. The rising nationalist and civil rights movements prompted essayist Harold Cruse to predict, in a 1962 piece, that "Afro-Americans . . . will undoubtedly make a lot of noise in militant demonstrations, cultivate beards and sport their hair in various degrees of *la mode au naturel*. . . ." One year later, Nigerian writer Theresa Ogunbiyi and associate editor of *Jet* Helen Hayes King copublished an article entitled "Should Negro Women Straighten Their Hair?" Although integrationists were very interested in looking visually acceptable to Whites, they were also showing Black people that it was okay to rise up, take a stand, and fight. The seeds of resistance that were planted in the young men and women who listened to the teachings of nationalists such as Malcolm X or participated in the Freedom Rides and sit-ins of the Civil Rights movement were to take root, eventually producing the leaders of the Black Power movement, leaders who demanded that Blacks redefine themselves visually in order to find true and total emancipation.

3

Revolutionary Roots: Naturals, Afros, and the Changing Politics of Hair, 1965–1979

Black Is Beautiful

In 1964 Philadelphia artist Samuel Roosevelt was an eighteen-year-old Air Force Airman First Class stationed in the Philippines. And he had a problem. After a number of fruitless searches and some unfortunate haircuts, Roosevelt was unable to find a good barber. His solution was simply to let his hair grow. Upon release from the military in 1966, Roosevelt and his uncut hair returned home to Philadelphia—where he was promptly made fun of by friends and family. "They told me that I looked a mess and needed to go and do my hair," Roosevelt recalls. "Then less than a year later they were running around with Afro picks, trying to get their 'fros higher and acting like that was how they had looked all of their lives."

Between 1964 and 1966, colored people and Negroes "became" Black people. And these Black people overwhelmingly chose to adopt a new, Black-identified visual aesthetic, an aesthetic that not only incorporated an alternative to straight hair but actually celebrated it.

In the mid-sixties, Black hair underwent its biggest change since Africans arrived in America. The very perception of hair shifted from one of style to statement. And right or wrong, Blacks and Whites came to believe that the way Black people wore their hair said something about their politics. Hair came to symbolize either a continued move toward integration in the American political system or a growing cry for Black power and nationalism. Many African-Americans began to use their hair as a way to show a visible connection to their African ancestors and Blacks throughout the diaspora. It was an era in which hair took a prime spot—right next to placards, amendments, and marches—in defining a Black identity for the world at large.

In 1966, when First Class Airman Roosevelt went back to Philadelphia, the political situation in Black America was growing increasingly more volatile. Key Black leaders were dead, including Medgar Evers and Malcolm X. The Black Power movement was taking shape. In light of the continued advances of the Civil Rights movement, such as the passage of the 1963 Voting Rights Act, the stark inequalities in the very fabric of the American social system came into clearer view for many Blacks. So as integrationists such as Martin Luther King Jr. and his Southern Christian Leadership Council (SCLC) continued to push for greater inclusion into mainstream society, another contingent of Blacks came to push for something different—a strengthened Black world, one that encompassed politics, economics, art, literature, education, and a new aesthetic.

A new way of defining beauty may seem an unlikely tenet for a revolutionary movement. But for Blacks in America, a new way of looking at themselves was as revolutionary as most anything could be. They had been more than three hundred years in a land that had collectively stripped them of pride in their Blackness—including pride in the color of their skin and all distinctly African physical attributes. In time many Blacks came to dismiss these characteristics as inferior. "We had been completely brainwashed and we didn't even know it. We accepted White value systems and White standards of beauty and, at times, we accepted the White man's view of ourselves," Assata Shakur, former Black Panther, explains in her autobiography. "We had never been exposed to any other point of view or any other standard of beauty."

A people wanting to assert their pride and unity needed to have pride in how they looked. The first major move was to embrace the very word *Black*. Prior to the mid-sixties, the word *Black* had only negative connotations. As Assata Shakur remembers in her autobiography, "Black made any insult worse. In fact, when I was growing up, being called 'Black' period, was grounds for fighting. We would talk about each other's ugly, big lips and flat noses. We would call each other 'pickaninnies' and nappy-haired so-and-so's." To be told that your hair was nappy was akin to having someone talk about your mama. Small children, mirroring the attitudes they were taught at home or in school, taunted one another with the rhyme "If you're White, you're all right, if you're Black, get back, if you're brown, stick around." Reporter and author Jill Nelson analogizes that in the early sixties the word *Black* carried the same connotations as *nigger*.

The shift to calling oneself Black and being proud of it translated into a style that proudly hearkened back to Africa. More than skin color, the word became a political statement in terms of one's consciousness, color, and culture. After generations of trying to neutralize distinctive African characteristics, people began to celebrate them. And just as hair had been central to the way Blacks of earlier years had sought to mainstream themselves, hair became a key determinant in visually declaring Black Pride. Marcia Gillespie, editor-in-chief of *Ms.* magazine and former editor of *Essence* magazine, reasons that "Being on the [slave] ship, not being able to comb [the hair], being shackled and sold, must have made Blacks feel so debased. The Afro was like a journey to reclaim ourselves from that."

"After the sit-ins, Freedom Rides, Watts and Selma, we took a good look at ourselves and while everyone was watching we bared our souls," wrote beauty culturist Lois Liberty Jones in *All About the Natural*, a popular how-to book of the time. "We found our Black beauty and the pride to go with it." In the mid-sixties not only was there a move to use the word *Black* in self-description, but many African-Americans sought to make blackness beautiful. Those three simple words "Black is beautiful" were first uttered during the 1960s. At first part of a larger political manifesto, Black beauty overwhelmingly translated to wearing African-derived dress, such as dashikis, and most significantly, the Afro hairstyle.

Black artists, such as Faith Ringgold, used their different mediums to explore the politics of beauty and an African-based beauty ideal. Some artists used their actual hair as an expression of art. Singer Abbey Lincoln, who began wearing her hair unstraightened in the late 1950s, explained, "I discovered at the time that my hair was my crown, so I wore it naturally." While for some, art was celebration, others used it to teach and encourage Black Americans to question their beliefs. In 1966 Nina Simone released "Four Women," a song about Black women of varying skin tones and hair textures that questioned ideas of beauty and the connection between these ideas and self-acceptance and love. Although it was banned on a number of Black radio stations because some deemed it insulting, "Four Women" was meant to shake Black women up into accepting themselves as they visually were.

The Birth of a Hairstyle

As with all things Black, the Afro's roots lie in Africa, though incidentally, not in the regions of the continent where America's first slaves were captured. In the late fifties and early sixties, it was popular among South African women to wear their hair in small "bushes," another name for the Afro. At this same time, a contingent of artists and intellectuals based in New York's Greenwich Village stopped straightening their hair. Women such as Nina Simone, Abbey Lincoln, and the folksinger Odetta were part of this group, and each of them embraced natural hair and traditional African cornrowed styles.

A New York hairdresser named Camello Casimir, better known as Frenchie, helped introduce naturally textured Black hair to the mainstream after cutting South African singer Miriam Makeba's hair in a short 'fro for the January 1960 issue of *Look* magazine. In 1962 Cicely Tyson appeared on the CBS drama series *East Side, West Side* with her hair in an Afro and, in subsequent episodes, in cornrows. Yet it was not until roughly four years later that the Afro started to become more commonplace as college students adopted it. Soon well-known Afroed Black political and cultural figures, such as political activist and future presidential candidate Jesse Jackson, were on the picket lines fighting for injustice. "When we started wearing dashikis and our Afros, we made a huge political statement," recalls Jackson in Lloyd Boston's *Men of Color*. "I feel that the way

I wore my hair was an expression of the rebellion of the time. It was our first statement which was not easy to imitate."

While not every Black American adopted the Afro (in fact, the chemical straightening industry was alive and well), it is true that nearly all were affected or influenced by it. Generational conflicts developed with Black parents, grandparents, and clergymen who thought their children's appearance was an unforgivable disgrace. The Black hair-care industry, from beauticians to product manufacturers, was forced to reckon with a style that rendered its goods and services unnecessary. Young adults who did not adopt natural hair were now, for the first time in Black American history, being judged harshly and publicly by many of their peers for their decision to wear straight, "neat" hair.

As with many social revolutions, this aesthetic uprising took root on college campuses. It started in the mid-sixties with students who were reading the works of nationalist thinkers of the past, such as W. E. B. DuBois and Marcus Garvey, and with young men and women who were following the wars for independence that were being fought throughout Africa against imperialist European nations. Influenced and/or inspired by the nationalistic teachings of the Nation of Islam, these students became disillusioned with a culture that said the only path to success was through assimilation into mainstream White society. Soon some of these young adults, people like Kathleen Cleaver, Angela Davis, and Stokely Carmichael, who had perhaps once marched for the right to vote or participated in sit-ins, were on the nightly news, in *The New York Times*, and eventually even on the FBI's Most Wanted list—fist in the air, hair bushy and high—as leaders of the Black Power movement. The hairstyles they wore spread in popularity to entertainers such as Sly Stone, Jimi Hendrix, and Stevie Wonder. Soon it spread to the masses and even captured the attention of James Brown, who in 1969 released an anthem for the era called "I'm Black and I'm Proud" and, for a short period, unconked his press-and-curled 'do and sported unstraightened hair.

The Afro's message was about "freeing your mind," as explained in *All About the Natural*. "It's about a hairstyle that lets you say, 'I've got my own beauty with my sisters and my brothers.' . . . It is a hairstyle on its way to being a lifestyle. It says, 'look at us as we are, because that's how it is.' Simply put, it is a matter of reclaiming our soul." While such a declaration is a bit extreme in all that it expects a hairstyle to deliver, the Afro did offer countless Blacks an exciting, affirming alternative. Stationed at the time on a U.S. Army base in Germany, Specialist Fifth Class James Solomon remembers that in 1968, "I began to see magazine pictures of people with these *big* Afros. You can't imagine what it was like when you were brought up all your life to think something is your primary aesthetic and then you see the cover of *Ebony* with this person with puffed-out nappy hair. It was a strange feeling because part of me was like 'Should I like this?' and the other part of me said, 'Boy, I really like this!' It was like a natural super-charge." Reflecting now on that "supercharge," Solomon says that the style was "more than anything else, representing the opening of information of what Black people were doing."

Upon returning home and entering Pennsylvania's all-Black Cheyney University, twenty-year-old Solomon traded in his short army cut for an Afro. "It was 1969 and I was reading different literature, all kinds of stuff. It was a period of time where we were trying to find things out. We were modeling ourselves after people that were making those statements." The "statements" that he refers to were the foundations of the Black Power movement, and its leaders were people like H. Rap Brown, Huey Newton, Angela Davis, and Stokely Carmichael.

The Black Power movement had gained a substantial following and an even larger number of sympathizers by 1969. One year earlier, in a speech that launched a cultural revolution, Stokely Carmichael invoked the words *Black Power*. For lack of any other cohesive nationalist movement, all things that fell under the general heading of Black pride came to be attributed—by the media, White America, and other Blacks—to the work of the organization called the Black Panthers. So while the Panthers were actually more con-cerned with Head Start programs and challenging legal injustices, there was a growing legion of primarily younger Black Americans who were 'froing their hair in emulation of the Panthers and as a declaration of their racial pride. A student at Texas Southern University in the late sixties, Stanley Williams re-members that he first "saw [the Afro] on Black Panthers. I thought of it as a militant thing. It was about identity and being proud of being Black."

When Assata Shakur, still going by her birth name of JoAnne Chesimard, entered Manhattan Community College, she felt an awakening of both her political views and her self-image. "My image of myself was changing, as well as my concept of beauty. One day a friend asked me why I didn't wear my hair in an Afro, natural. . . . The more I thought about it the better it sounded. . . . To make [my hair] natural I literally had to cut the conk off," she wrote in her memoirs. "I cut it myself and then stood in the shower for hours melting the conk out. At last, my hair was free. On the subway, people stared at me, but my friends at school were supportive and encouraging."

Police captain Craig Price remembers that his primary reason for wearing an Afro "was to differentiate myself from Whites." For many like Price, who grew up during the forties and fifties when there was no public debate over conformity to a White aesthetic, the Afro allowed them the opportunity to voice their rejection consciously. "I had been made to wear my [pre-Afro] hair so short-cropped because of White people," continues Price. "It was all about conforming to look like [them]. Afros were the first time that Whites could look at you and collectively think, this person doesn't go along with my philosophy and doesn't care that I know."

And Afros were not the only way that unstraightened, nappy hair was being celebrated and worn. In fact, many of those now described as having worn an Afro were in fact wearing another look, one called the Natural. The Natural was unstraightened Black hair that was not cut close. It was a less sculpted, less maintained version of the rounded, perfectly actualized Afro. This mass of bushy, springy hair opened the door to endless styling possibilities. While styles for Black men were typically short-cropped or mile-high, Black women in record numbers began to experiment with creative styles that were meant for naturally textured Black hair. Afros of varying heights, cornrows, braids, and African-inspired headwraps, called gelées, gained popularity.

The ideological shifts signaled by the Afro were not solely about loving a Black aesthetic. "It wasn't just a look early on. It was a lot more political. There was some expectation toward your behavior, particularly your behavior toward other Black people, women, your brother," stresses Rochelle Nichols Solomon, Philadelphia education reformer and founding member of the community group Sisters Remember Malcolm. Whether the assessment was true or not, it was generally believed that one's hairstyle was indicative of one's politics. Hair straightening for both men and women, once considered a requirement for success, came to be read by many as the most obvious marker of one's attempts to emulate Whiteness. Now that Black was beautiful, straightening one's hair in the image of White beauty was seen as blasphemy.

The rhetoric and ideals of the time were rigid ones, as Marcia Gillespie explains: "This blacker than thou game, it started in the sixties. At first when people saw Afros they were like 'Why would they do *that*?' Then as the sixties got going, it was the bigger the better. If you didn't have a 'fro as big as Angela Davis or Kathleen Cleaver, it was like 'How black are you?' Or if you continued to straighten your hair, you got a lot of true-nationalistic-do-right-sister pressure." "An activist with straight hair was a contradiction, a lie, a joke really," wrote Gloria Wade-Gayles. Simply put, "You were an Uncle Tom," says former airman Roosevelt.

There were quite a few Black activists who cautioned against the moral policing that was taking place over hair. As far back as 1963, some warned that "folks tend to make too much of a connection between natural hair and liberation politics." But by 1969 those warnings had gone largely unheeded. In an article that appeared in a theme issue of *Ebony* magazine on the "Black Revolution," professor Charles V. Hamilton, coauthor (with Stokely Carmichael) of the book *Black Power*, wrote that an overemphasis and narrow defining of Blackness was leading to "increased confusion and danger [of] a game of trying to 'out-Black' or 'out-militant' one another. In some circles, one is not 'Black enough' unless one wears a dashiki, gives the Black power handshake and gets an Afro haircut." Hamilton stressed that these things were merely symbols of "the new awareness" among African-Americans and did not necessarily relate to "the *substance* of what the struggle [was] about." African-American author John O. Killens even created a fictitious, satirical "world championship of blackness contest" in his novel *The Cotillion* to highlight the pervasive issue.

College campuses, where the style first spread, also became a common site for this "blacker than thou" policing. "Nobody had straight hair," declares Rochelle Nichols Solomon about the politically active students on Cheyney University's campus in the late sixties. "The [people] that had naturally straight hair went and put chemicals in their hair to get it to nap up." For some African-Americans, rhetoric or no, growing an Afro simply was not possible. As a group, African-Americans have more hair textures than shades of complexion. Some Blacks were simply born without nappy hair. The sought-after "good hair" of the recent past was now a badge of shame for many. For others it may not have been a shame, but it was definitely a hindrance to getting the look they wanted.

While it may seem to go against the very ideas behind a style called

Natural to chemically kink your hair into an Afro, for many *not* having a 'fro was akin to being a race traitor. "Bad hair became good; good hair became a badge of miscegenating forebears, a difficult cross to bear," wrote Jill Nelson in a 1987 *Washington Post* article. "My loose-curled hair had once been 'good' but was now 'bad.' . . . I had to have a natural. . . . [I] couldn't face another minute of scorn from brothers in dashikis and sisters with gelées wrapped around their Afros." After a frustrating search for a solution, Nelson found a Harlem barber who suggested that she cut her hair short and then wash it in Octagon laundry soap. Inexplicably this worked, and she became a proud, card-carrying member of the Afroed masses.

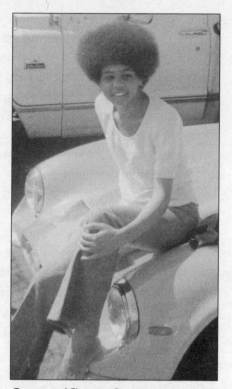

Courtesy of Florence Price.

Always a creative people when faced with obstacles, Blacks looking to "nap up" their hair to get an Afro found solutions. Celebrity hairstylist Mr. Andrews, who opened his New York City business in the 1960s, remembers, "I've had Black people with straight hair who wanted an Afro. So I invented a process. I would perm their straight hair nappy. It was a curly relaxer with perm rods—a simulated Afro. I got a lot of business doing that." Others relied on home concoctions, some of the most popular ingredients being vinegar, beer, and Borax cleanser.

Pride and Prejudice

Not everyone heralded the Afro as a change for the better. In fact, many viewed this purported reclamation of culture, identity, and an African-centered aesthetic quite unfavorably. Afros were not just a simple Black statement that "we are not straightening our hair in conformity to a Eurocentric ideal." They were an over-the-top expression—the higher the hair and the more it didn't look like anything that could be considered White, the better. And for many Whites, Afros—and all that they seemed to represent—inspired fear. Bernice Calvin, founder of the first Black hair trade show, stresses, "The Afro was a big, wild, striking thing. It actually frightened mainstream America because it was so much more radical that what they had been used to. It was the whole thought that [Blacks] were quiet for so long and all of sudden they got demanding."

For the first time since slavery and the days of the minstrel shows, White people were taking collective notice of how African-Americans wore their hair. And not all liked what they saw. Until the mid-sixties and the emergence of Afros and cornrows, Black hair showdowns (long versus short, nappy versus wavy, straight versus unstraight) had been waged *within* the Black community. Schools were segregated. So were most neighborhoods. There were precious few Blacks on television shows. There were no music videos. White Americans were not exposed to constant, evolving images of Blacks in popular culture, the arena in which most Americans encounter other groups. Now Black hair—unstraightened, bushy Black hair—was on the nightly news, attached to a man or woman making political demands that until then had never been voiced.

Initial mainstream disapproval of the Afro was definitely race-based, but hair had also become a contested issue in the political landscape of the sixties outside the Black community. It was the visual ground over which hippies, Black militants, and feminists battled it out with the "establishment." As captured by the play *Hair*, both Whites and Blacks at that time were growing their hair. "The establishment had their hair cut neat," recalls Samuel Roosevelt. "The Afro said that I was gonna wear my damn knotty hair as long as I want." So in characterizing the liberal mood of the day, Blacks with Afros took their place alongside White "longhairs."

Conflicts over hair and the Afro were also being fought within the Black community. While the sixties and seventies have now been freeze-framed in history as a time when all Blacks happily embraced Afros and natural hair, there were many who rejected or wholeheartedly disapproved of the style. This division often cut across regional and generational lines. While some parents and older African-Americans saw Afros simply as an expression of youth, similar to their own zoot suits and jazz, many others disapproved. Florence Price, a septuagenarian grandmother of four, thought

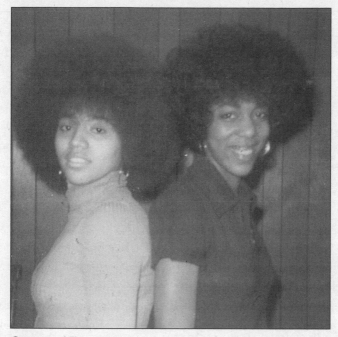

Courtesy of Florence Price.

that Afros "were just a disgrace. My daughter and son had Afros *out to here.* I just didn't like 'em. They didn't do anything for the person wearing them." Some parents were dead set against the idea of their children wearing a Bush. "My friend," Price continues, "went to pick her daughter up who was coming home from college and she had grown an Afro. My friend just stood there in that airport, looking at her daughter, and screamed." One woman who grew up in 1960s Milwaukee said, "I wanted to go natural like all of my friends, and my mother was totally enraged. She told me if I was going to let my hair go natural I would have to go back to the jungle. To my mother it was like I was contemplating not bathing."

Other reactions were even more negative. Seventeen-year-old Rochelle Nichols unknowingly declared a battle of wills with her mother when she stopped straightening her hair in 1967. What began as an innocent expression of her changing politics turned into a summer of Nichols's mother leaving notes on the front door that read "No Afros allowed in this house," notes that prompted her daughter to take up temporary residence at the local YWCA. "My mother and my fights were about hair, but it was more than that," explains Nichols Solomon. "It was about my growing up and my politics and deciding things on my own. Above my bed, after one of our fights, I hung this poem that I wrote. It went, 'When I die I will be happy. Because Jesus will love me with my hair nappy.'"

Within Black communities across the country, significant segments would have given just about anything to see the return of straight hair. "A lot of people had negative reactions to the Afro because they were raised a different way," reasons James Solomon. "It was almost like there was a hysteria to a look and to an idea." For some, Afros were an aesthetic horror. After a lifetime of believing that hair was meant to be straight, glossy, and neat, they found the extremism of the Afro unpalatable. Cicely Tyson recalled in *Jet* magazine how the harshest critics of the braids and cornrows that she wore on her CBS series were other Black people, who "were irate because they felt that I was portraying a negative image of the Black woman."

Parents and older generation African-Americans were not the only ones who disapproved of the style. Many average folks just did not care for the politics behind the style. For the Black church, a long-standing pillar of the community, disapproval of the Afro was not based on its aesthetics but was typically a condemnation of all that the look represented ideologically. While the Civil Rights movement had politicized many ministers and congregation members, the Black church was still overwhelmingly conservative. In the burgeoning years of the Black Power movement, the church was generally not a major supporter of the rising militancy. This carried through to the issue of hair. Dr. Cheryl Ajirotutu, a professor of anthropology at the University of Wisconsin who grew up in Oakland, California, at the height of that city's Black militant activity, remembers Sundays at her church: "I went to Baptist church, and every week the minister would make everyone with an Afro stand up and tell us we were all going to hell." Though this response is extreme, such outrage did exist. While many Blacks supported the ideas behind the Black Power movement, others found it to be reactionary, aggressive, and negative. Black Midwesterner Juanita Bradford, who was a teenager at the time, remembers, "I was afraid of Afros, dashikis, and guys that looked and acted like H. Rap Brown. I thought Afros were negative. I never thought of them as beautiful or positive or powerful. I saw them as violent, militant, and separatist. I guess I was a bit ashamed of them."

For some the reasons for disliking the Afro were less personal and instead about the almighty dollar. Hairdressers in particular were averse to the style. Many believed it was going to ruin their business as people switched to the services offered by barbers and significantly fewer women desired press-and-curls. Black hair-product manufacturers faced a recession, as many customers who had once depended on hot combs, relaxer kits, pomades, and curlers no longer needed them. It would take a few years after the initial appearance of the style in the mid-sixties for manufacturers to adjust and develop Afro- and natural-hair-specific products.

The Growing Depoliticization of Hair: 1971–1979

In March 1971, the one-year-old Black women's magazine *Essence* hit newsstands with its first-ever cover model with long, straight hair. Its past issues had all featured Afroed or cornrowed cover subjects. The model's name was Lauren Walker, and she was not a professional model but instead a "new breed . . . one of the many up-and-coming business-minded women of the future."

Walker's professed business-mindedness in a youth and popular culture that had just recently invested the bulk of its interest in revolution was as startling as her hairstyle. But by 1971 the Black Power movement was losing momentum, and Black hair's natural reign was undergoing a change. The Afro had become a hairstyle, plain and simple. It was no longer a matter of what your 'fro stood for but of how high your 'fro stood. Afros were everywhere, and they were increasingly unconnected to Black Power. Younger adults, who were coming of age after the Civil Rights movement, began wearing the style in emulation of celebrities like Jimi Hendrix rather than activists like Angela Davis. The Jackson 5, a group few would argue were pushing any type of subversive political agenda, had mile-high Afros. Diana Ross, the epitome of mainstream appeal, even sported a short Bush. White people, now used to the style that had shocked them just a few short years before, were beginning to co-opt it. And Blacks, now used to the style and increasingly forgetful of its ideological meanings, were like Whites, reinterpreting it simply as a hairstyle that could be worn today and gone tomorrow.

White America became more at ease with the sight of a large Afro at roughly the same time that the Black Power movement was losing most of its steam. Internal dissonance, caused or exacerbated by government sabotage as well as trumped-up criminal charges and government-endorsed acts of terrorism, led the Black Panthers and similar militant groups to fall apart. Many who had been part of the Black Power movement abandoned it. "The cause died," notes Stephanie Williams, a former Panther sympathizer whose own Afro had been inspired by H. Rap Brown. "The Afro became a fashion statement."

The Afro's shift from statement to style was in some ways necessary in the continued move for an increased Black consciousness. The hairstyle had perhaps been given too much meaning, diverting attention from other necessary aspects of revolution and change. The screening process for a revolutionary had come to depend too much on his or her Afro pick. "People are right when they say it's not what you have on your head but what you have in it," wrote Shakur in her autobiography. "You can be a revolutionary-thinking person and have your hair fried up. And you can have an Afro and be a traitor to Black people." Author and professor Carolivia Herron remembers her reasons for keeping her own hair straight during the height of Howard University's Black militant activity. "When I was at Howard and everyone was going natural with Afros, I refused to do it because I wanted to show that I could be just as radical as they were without it being in my hair. I actually preferred Afros, but I didn't do it to show that people could rob you and cheat you with an Afro two feet high. Wearing an Afro didn't mean you had your soul in the right place."

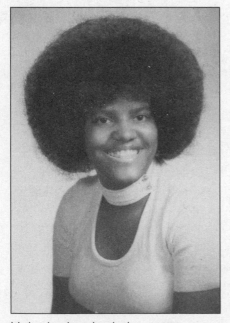

High school yearbook photo, 1974. Courtesy of Florence Price.

In certain ways the Afro, the symbol of Black Beauty, had achieved its goals by the middle of the seventies. As it became, to the lament of many who still pushed a Black Power agenda, *just* a hairstyle, at the very least it became a hairstyle that demanded an alternative, African-derived aesthetic be recognized and heralded. In some ways America had appeared to enlarge its defini-

Nat "The Bush Doctor" Mathis Speaks

I opened my first shop in April 1, 1969, when I was twenty-three. It was called Nat's Hair Care Clinic. When Afros first came out, people were just wearing them natural and it put a lot of people out of work. There were a lot of "For Sale" signs. A lot of barbershops didn't know how to style it. You have to learn how to read hair like you read a book. So I was thinking, how could I get people to get their hair shampooed, not just a haircut, but to get them to shampoo it, condition it, blow it out, trim it, and style it. The idea I was focusing on was to treat the hair, not just cut it.

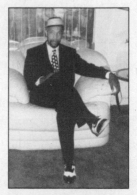

Nat "The Bush Doctor" Mathis. Courtesy of Nathaniel Mathis.

So I took it to the schools—elementary and junior high. I had this guy called the Mechanical Man and we had a skit where I had an announcer and he would come out and talk to the kids, give them a little pep talk and then introduce me and I would do hairstyles. We had strobe lights, and I would be styling hair and the Mechanical Man was dancing.

I got the name Bush Doctor because I called myself the Hair Doctor. Then when the Afro came out and I started styling it, the neighborhood started calling me the Bush Doctor. And then the name really stuck when I did this TV program as a publicity stunt for my business. In 1970 there was a local disc jockey who had a radio and TV show. I got on his program and did a White woman's hair—long blond straight hair—and made it into an Afro.

At the time you had different groups of people who were wearing the Afro. My look at the time was an Afro with a part in the middle. You had conservative people who just wore it because it was a fad. And you had people protesting the war who wore it. Then you had people protesting segregation and groups like the Black Panthers. Their hair was a part of that. But I think the Afro started out with people like Frederick Douglass. It has always been around and always will be.

People always ask me, Why haven't you changed your name? Why are you still the Bush Doctor? Well, really, if you think about it, even when people get relaxers and they have new hair grow out, it's still an Afro up under there. And I'm just doctoring the hair. I'm a doctor.

tion of what was beautiful or at least acceptable. The army and numerous airlines had gone so far as to change their uniform hats to accommodate bushy, natural Black hair. Marcia Gillespie, who served as editor-in-chief of *Essence* magazine in 1975, remembers, "What we [at *Essence*] tried to do was show the rainbow. And readers really wanted to see themselves and the range of black beauty. That everyone is beautiful." *Essence* was the first to fill its pages with stories and photo layouts of wigs (including Afro wigs), weaves, hairpieces, and straight styles alongside styles for natural hair. The visual alternative that the Black Power movement and a legion of Black Americans had put forth was now apparent in many avenues of Black and mainstream society. High school and college yearbooks were filled with the faces of Afroed and cornrowed Black youth and young adults. On television, Black female characters such as Thelma on *Good Times* were sex symbols, but more importantly they were visual examples to other Black women of Black beauty accepted by a mass society.

The mid-1970s ushered in one of the biggest sex symbols of American popular culture. She had a huge Afro and was idolized by Whites as well as Blacks. Her name was Pam Grier, and she was the star of blaxploitation films including *Foxy Brown* and *Coffy*. Grier's pop culture significance goes beyond pinup status, as she is credited by many with popularizing the Afro for Blacks. A 1997 *InStyle* magazine article on the century's most important hairstyles notes that in 1974 Grier "pulled a gun from her mighty Afro" and made the look a fashion statement. *Washingtonian* magazine applauded the actress for giving Black women a "proud, natural style" in an article on "Great Moments in Hair." Statements such as the *Washingtonian*'s not only push forward the date of the style by more than a decade but also take it out of any political context.

Blaxploitation films and their stars not only helped to remove any sociopolitical meaning from the fashions and styles they highlighted but also exaggerated many negative facets of Black life, including drug dealing, pimping, and golddigging women. These hyperbolized images were not being swapped in the barbershops and pool halls of Black neighborhoods but instead were offered as visual consumption for a White audience. The effect of films such as *Shaft*, *Superfly*, and *Cleopatra Jones* on Black hair was that, at the most extreme, it placed the Afro in the midst of buffoonery. At the very least, it normalized the style and placed it so far out of any context of Black revolution and pride (though some of these films did have pseudo–Black nationalist plotlines) that Whites who had once felt intimidated could now relax when an Afro passed their way.

One of the most popular films of this era, *Superfly*, featuring the über-coiffed Ron O'Neal, spawned its own hairstyle, named after its smooth-talking, smoother-haired star. By 1973 Black men around the country were paying up to twenty-five dollars to get their hair permed and then curled in the Superfly, a bouffant style similar to the look still worn by singer James Brown. The style required a tremendous amount of hair, indicating that the men who had enough hair to wear it had previously had Afros. These men traded in their emulation of revolutionaries for the look of a fictitious pimp and drug dealer.

For those Blacks who still wore an Afro, the hairstyle itself was changing. It now came with its own new set of beauty demands. During the early days of the style, men and women often cornrowed and plaited their hair at night in order to have a looser, higher Afro in the morning. But as the style became more visible in everyday walks of life, and as models such as Peggy Dillard wore it on runways around the world, the Afro became regimented, as many aspects of beauty culture are. A book on how to care for natural hair stressed, "We can all wear the [Afro], but remember at its best it is not a do-it-yourself thing. There is the 'primitive' Natural and there's the well-groomed coiffure."

Not coincidentally, this raising of visual standards happened at the same time the Black hair-care industry figured out how to inch into the Afro market. In the late sixties, an Afro pick was the only tool deemed necessary for upkeep. But soon after, beauty manufacturers found a way to make money from the look, and Afro Sheen and various other glycerin-based products were introduced, promoted as softeners intended to make the hair more manageable. There were even packages, called blowout kits, that contained a mild relaxer and were sold to loosen the hair's natural kink and maximize the volume that the Afro could reach. George Great-house, owner of the Esquire Barber Shop, the professed site of Phoenix, Arizona's first Afro haircut, told a reporter that "the secret to the 'fro was air supplied by a blow-dryer. A long-toothed comb was used to lift the hair away from the scalp. An application of glycerin kept the hair from being torched by the dryer's intense heat." Softer hair was "shaped up" with scissors and then clippers were used to achieve the ideal rounded shape. Numerous hair historians, such as Lloyd Boston, note the sad contradiction

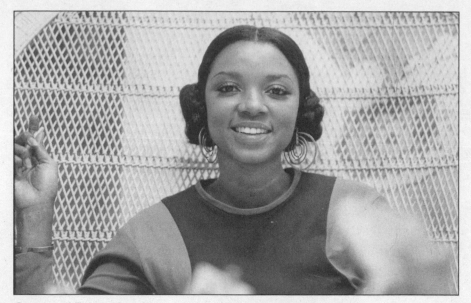

Courtesy of Florence Price.

of the style's original intentions that was evident in these products, which were designed to promise a "better" Afro by straightening the hair.

By the mid-seventies, many major Black leaders were dead, exiled, or in jail, Pam Grier was in Hollywood, and Barbra Streisand had an Afro. Yet and still, for some Blacks the reason for getting rid of the Afro was less dramatic and more pragmatic. Many brothers and sisters of the revolution had to get a job. With drastic cutbacks in state and federal aid to cities and social programs, many of the jobs available to people who had stayed on the fringe of the mainstream were now shutting down. It was time for many to go to work with "the Man," and as in the past the Man most often required a "well-groomed" haircut. James Solomon, now married and the father of two, explains cutting his hair down in 1975: "I started looking for another job. I didn't care. I felt as though the aesthetic had served its purpose in terms of letting people know there's something else out there. But as far as personal style, I cut my hair because it was an expression of what I needed to do."

The Afro and other natural hairstyles were disappearing into the background, as captured in a 1977 *Washington Post* piece called "The Afro Doing a Graceful Fadeout." Sales figures for relaxer kits were on the rise. Some attributed it simply to Black women wanting a new style and more flexibility in how to wear their hair. Others believed that natural hair had never really been accepted by some and that straight hair had always remained, lurking in the background, as the desired look. "I know a lot of sisters who got naturals so that they'd be more attractive so that they could get a man," reasons Rochelle Nichols Solomon, who today keeps her unstraightened hair cut short. "They embraced certain aspects of revolutionary thought to be with these brothers. So when the seventies came and things started changing, sisters that I thought I shared a vision with, about not hair so much as a lifestyle and way of thinking, they were throwing it off. Going for the perms. I couldn't believe it. They never internalized it."

As the 1980s loomed on the horizon, America was changing. Conservatism was replacing the liberal mood that had characterized much of the previous twenty years. A "me" mentality was chipping away at the communal unity that had supported much of the social change and revolutionary movements of the recent past. After nearly two decades of amendments, marches, and protests, Black America was not only without a collective leader but still earning less and generally worse off than the average White citizen. In many ways it would seem as if the fight for equality and self-determination should still be under way. But it was not. While the Afro and natural hair may have forced a broadening of the idea of what was considered beautiful and proud, in many ways victory was declared too soon. The United States was two hundred years old, and for the duration of its history Blacks and their features had been deemed ugly. It would take more than a few years and a few Afros to turn things around. "Maybe in another time, when everybody is equal and free, it won't matter how anybody wears their hair or dresses or looks," predicted Assata Shakur in the pages of her autobiography. "There won't be any oppressors to mimic or avoid mimicking." Until then, however, Black hair was returning to business as usual.

4

The Business of
Black Hair

The House of the Lord Pentecostal Church stands on Atlantic Avenue, surrounded by antique stores and Middle Eastern restaurants near downtown Brooklyn. A simple limestone structure with a massive red door and weathered stained-glass windows, it is an especially popular location for funerals. It was a bitter winter day in February 1987 when the Lord Pentecostal was home to one of the most well-attended funerals in the church's history. Over four hundred African-American mourners were in attendance, including civic leaders and politicians—all vying for a view of the massive pine coffin. Interestingly enough there was no corpse in the coffin, but the people gathered were prepared for death—death to Revlon, Incorporated.

This mock funeral was actually one of over forty protests supported by the Reverend Jesse Jackson's social activist organization, Operation PUSH, against the cosmetic giant's imminent takeover of the ethnic (read Black or kinky) hair industry. Furthermore, Revlon executive Irving Bottner had recently made the tactless blunder of bragging about the company's success in the African-American hair-care market in *Newsweek* magazine, saying, "In the next couple of years, the Black-owned businesses will disappear. They'll all be sold to White companies." Tossing hundreds of Revlon bottles into the coffin and vowing to bury Revlon with a boycott of their products, African-American protesters made it clear they would not stand by and allow "the Man" to take over an industry that had been a source of pride, achievement, and economic empowerment since the beginning of the Black experience in America. Right or wrong, when it comes to the business of hair, Black people get fiercely protective.

Freedom and Riches in the Barbershops and Salons of America: 1700–1800

Before the Civil War, contrary to popular belief, not all Black people spent their lives picking cotton on a plantation down South. There were an estimated fifty thousand free Blacks in the North American British colonies in the early eighteenth century. By the beginning of the next century that number, according to census reports, increased to 108,435. Whether free from birth or recently manumitted, Blacks were employed in almost every field—law, education, real estate, medicine, banking—and often owned their own businesses. One of the most lucrative enterprises for free Black men at this early stage in America's history was owning a barbershop that catered exclusively to White clients.

The Black-owned barbershops of this era provided a haven for the pampered Caucasian elite, offering public baths and spa and beauty treatments as well as barbering and hairdressing services. One Black-owned Saint Louis barbershop and bathhouse advertised such amenities as "recently installed baths with tubs of the finest Italian marble [and] rooms large, airy and elegantly furnished." Noted historian Juliet E. Walker, author of *The History of Black Business in America*, found that Black barbers dominated the antebellum barbering industry because they "invest[ed] their profits in providing state-of-the art services in elegant shops for their clients." Before the Civil War, it was the Black barbers who were setting the trends in the hair-care and bath services field. "The most fashionable coiffeur" in the city of New York in the eighteenth century was a former slave named Pierre Toussant. After buying his freedom and tending to the cosmetic needs of some of the finest French families in the city, he became one of the country's first Black philanthropists, donating much of his money to the Catholic Church. John B. Vashon, a Black Pittsburgh barber, opened the first public city bathhouse west of the Alleghenies in 1820. Frank Parrish, a Black barbershop and bathhouse owner, prospered for twenty years by offering his male and female clients "the luxury of the falling spray and the coolness of the flood" at his Nashville bathhouse, where he also sold specialty items like "fancy soaps, perfumes, cigars and tobacco."

The financial rewards were so great for Black barbers that many used their earnings to buy property, donate to charity, and establish additional businesses. William W. Watson, a Cincinnati barber and a former slave, had an estimated worth of thirty thousand dollars in the mid-1800s. Watson used his earnings to free his mother and siblings from slavery and to contribute large sums to the building of Black churches. North Carolina barber John Stanley, the son of a White father and an African mother, opened his own barbershop and amassed a great fortune that included sixty-four of his own slaves (he eventually freed eighteen of them, including his wife and children). Lewis Woodson, a Pittsburgh barber and minister, partnered with fellow barber John Vashon to cofound Wilberforce University, the first all-Black university. Almost across the board, antebellum Black barbers used their resources to help promote the development of the Black community at large. Sadly, these same barbers were unable or unwilling to cater to members of their own race for fear of their White clients' defection. In his 1818 *Sketches of America*, British writer Henry Fearon "could scarcely conceal his amazement at the fact that any Black hairdresser who wished to retain his White clientele could not service a perfectly respectable-looking Black man."

In both the North and South, antebellum Black barbers carved a place for themselves among the social and economic elite of Black America. Barbershops were most often family-run, providing financial stability for future generations. Initially, however, free Black women were not very successful in the hair business because of the oppressive sexism and racism in early American society. Male barbers, therefore, were charged with serving both male and female clients. In fact, Black male émigrés from the French West Indies were in high demand as female hairstylists because of their supposed expertise with European fashion and style. While it was incredibly difficult for a woman of any color to open and operate an independent business, on a few occasions—in New Orleans especially—slave owners trained their female slaves in the art of hairdressing and then hired them out to style hair in the homes of wealthy White women. Of course these slave women rarely enjoyed any of the fruits of their labor.

Eventually, around the 1820s, free Black women began to make inroads as hair professionals, due in part to the increase in racial hostility felt around the country toward Black men. In the final decades before the Civil War, Black men were increasingly being maligned as violent and sexually aggressive by southern Confederates looking for reasons to justify the enslavement of the Negro race. Because of this collective character assassination, Black men were forbidden to perform so intimate a task as styling a White woman's hair. Free Black women, therefore, stepped up to the plate. New Orleans was considered the center of the hair-care industry for White women because the extreme weather conditions (sun, heat, humidity) made styling and treatments a daily necessity. Black women like one Eliza Potter capitalized on this factor and set up shop. For eleven years Potter styled the hair of her well-to-do White clients in Louisiana and supplemented her income by training plantation slaves to do the same. Within the plantation system, slaves who knew how to barber and style White hair were elevated in the slave hierarchy to just below butlers, maids, and cooks but far above the field slave. Some industrious Black women—free and slave—set up cottage industries, making hair ointments, tonics, and salves, from a mixture of plants, herbs, and natural oils, that were similar to the products made in Africa. A small number of free Black women turned their homes into beauty parlors for other Black women, styling hair as well as selling their homemade hair goods.

One aspect of the hair trade that Black women were able to enter successfully in antebellum America was wig making. Three Black sisters, Cecilia, Marchita, and Caroline Redmond, owned and operated the Ladies Wig Salon, the largest antebellum wig factory in the state of Massachusetts, as well as a popular beauty parlor. Catering primarily to a wealthy White clientele, the Redmond sisters made hairpieces from the hair their customers collected from their combs and brushes. For Black women, the sisters sold a hair-loss treatment called Mrs. Putnam's Medicated Hair Tonic. They eventually expanded into a mail-order business serving the entire New England area.

After the Civil War, between Reconstruction and the turn of the century, Black businessmen began to abandon the service industries, including barbershops that catered to wealthy Whites. A combination of Jim Crow segregation and new economic opportunities caused many Blacks to try their hands at new endeavors in support of the rising Black middle class. Undertaking, banking, and insurance captured the attention of skillful Black entrepreneurs. After 1870, the number and proportion of prosperous Black barbers dropped sharply from 10 percent to less than 1.7 percent of the Black economic elite.

Big Money in Black Hair: 1900–1950

The turn of the century ushered in the birth of a Black middle class with cash to spend. As Blacks migrated into the cities, both Black and White entrepreneurs created goods and services to exploit this growing market. Black men and women were finally provided with commercial hair products instead of having to rely on homemade and often ineffectual concoctions. These products, however, were mostly tins of grease and "magic potions," purported to turn short, kinky hair into long, straight, shiny locs. At the beginning of the century, most manufacturers of these products were White and did not succeed in turning a great profit, mainly because the products were both marketed ineffectively and never lived up to their hyperbolic claims. But things changed rather quickly. Black people rolled up their sleeves and once again reclaimed the hair industry, but this time it was their own hair that caused profits to soar.

The two heroines of this stage of explosive entrepreurship in hair care were women. Annie Turnbo Malone and Madam C. J. Walker proved to the world just how lucrative Black hair could be. Using a combination of marketing savvy, business acumen, and the psychology of "looking good," both these turn-of-the-century crusaders transformed misfortune into a financial fortune for themselves and countless others.

Regardless of who sold the first jar of Wonderful Hair Grower, what is truly significant about these two entrepreneurs is how they revolutionized the Black hair-care industry. Prior to their entrance into the market at the turn of the century, manufacturers of Black hair-care products were over-whelmingly White men. Two of the more successful White-owned com-panies targeting Blacks were Plough and Ozonized Ox Marrow. Their method of marketing products like hair growers and pomades was to prey on the insecurities of Black people, promising a cure for the curse of kinky hair. Advertisements from the time read like personal insults: "Race men and women may easily have straight, soft, long hair by simply applying Plough's Hair Dressing and in a short time all your kinky, snarly, ugly hair becomes soft, silky, smooth . . . ," read one such ad running in a 1910 New York newspaper. Another demeaning document appearing in 1905 for a product called Curl-I-Cure commented, "Positively nothing detracts so much from your appearance as short, matted un-attractive hair."

The truth of the matter was that many Black people, men and women, desired straight hair, but the insulting ad copy used by White hair-care manufacturers left Black consumers wary and angered. In fact, the general sentiment within the Black community was that these White-owned com-panies were probably selling hair-care and cosmetic products that would prove harmful, maybe even deadly, to the Negro race. The controversy was followed closely by the Black press. "Too many ads smack of antebellum-ism, disrespect and a low grade of intelligence," read an editorial in the national Black women's publication *Half Century Magazine*. Black newspaper editorials, like those found in the *Chicago-Whip*, warned readers not to trust "advertisements for dangerous preparations made by White men. Be beauti-ful if you can, but don't burn your brains out in the attempt." For Blacks at the turn of the century, something so simple as hairstyling had become fraught with political overtones, health risks, and issues of racial pride. The market, therefore, was ripe for an Annie Malone or Madam C. J. Walker to introduce a line of health and beauty products made by Black people for Black people. Both of these women knew firsthand the unique hair prob-lems Blacks faced in this era, like chronic hair loss and scalp diseases, and tailored their products to address them. The Walker company's bestsellers before 1920 included a sulfur-based Vegetable Shampoo that helped heal infected scalps and Wonderful Hair Grower.

It has been reported that Madam Walker copied the recipe for her Won-derful Hair Grower from Annie Malone's Poro Company, even though

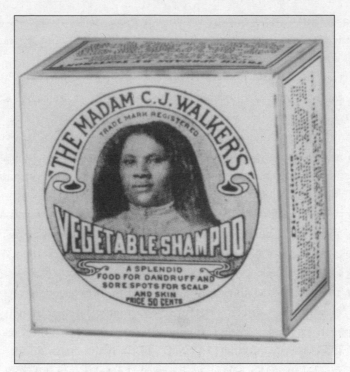

Madam C. J. Walker's Vegetable Shampoo. © A'Lelia Bundles,
Walker Family Collection, Alexandria, Virginia.

Walker herself claimed the ingredients came to her in a fantastical dream.
Coincidentally, Walker was living in Saint Louis, but had quit working as a
Poro agent when she had this dream. Before attempting to sell her "new"
hair grower, however, she moved to Denver, Colorado, so as not to clash
with Malone. "The formula [for the hair grower] was not new," confirms
biographer A'Lelia Bundles, who freely admits that her famous ancestor,
Madam Walker, probably used the same basic recipe as Malone's product
or any other alleged hair grower popular at the time. Bundles says that
anybody—with or without a background in chemistry—could have produced a batch of the stuff at home. "It's basically petrolatum, sulfur and
beeswax," Bundles discloses. Still, Walker's brand of Wonderful Hair Grower
was one of her best sellers because she knew how to market it by using her
own replenished locs as a testament to the product's effectiveness. An Atlanta woman wrote to Walker in 1917: "Dear Madam, When I began to use
your excellent Hair Preparations my hair was short and stubborn, but now it

is long and fluffy and I can dress it up in the current styles. I was almost baldheaded when I began to use your goods, so I cannot praise them enough. They are a Godsend to humanity."

The fact that Walker was a dark-complected woman with decidedly African features and a humble background helped solidify her earnest sales pitch. Black people were hungry for a product that worked but also for a manufacturer they could feel good about supporting. "It wasn't about the ingredients in the product," Bundles explains. "It was [Madam's] marketing genius and her personal charisma." White-owned companies were trying to sell shampoo and glossines using unrealistic, derogatory before-and-after depictions of Black women. Walker used before-and-after pictures of herself on her products, accompanied by her own inspirational story, to encourage others not only to purchase Walker products but to sell them as well.

Both Walker and Malone utilized a pyramid selling strategy, popularized in 1886 by the California Perfume Company (later known as Avon) to maximize their sales. Trained sales agents across the country would purchase Walker or Poro products in bulk and then sell them door-to-door. In a letter sent to her agents, Walker likened the sales strategy to a religious mission. "Keep in mind that you have something that the person standing before you really needs," she suggested. "Imagine yourself a missionary and convert him." The overwhelming majority of these door-to-door salespeople were low-income women who now had a chance at economic independence instead of a lifetime of domestic service or sharecropping. Compared with an unskilled White worker at this time, who earned about eleven dollars a week, a Walker agent was earning up to fifteen dollars a day. Malone and Walker also used incentive programs to motivate their agents. For example, at a Walker Beauty Culturists convention in 1918, the company gave a one-hundred-dollar cash prize to the agent who had signed up the most new agents. At Poro's peak around 1918, the company employed 240 staff members and boasted 68,000 sales agents nationwide. Walker arranged annual national conventions at which all her agents converged in one place to share ideas, socialize, and hear about new products and systems being developed by the company. Walker also established the first hairdresser's union for Black women. Both Walker and Malone established comprehensive beauty colleges where students became skilled beauticians and could then open a salon or style hair in the home using the official Walker or Poro system.

Madam C. J. Walker's most enduring legacy was not her door-to-door selling strategy, nor was it a single product. It was her method for straightening hair. Not content simply to sell hot combs, Walker marketed an entire hair-straightening process—known as the Walker system—that required a combination of her products to achieve maximum results. Available for purchase to trained Walker agents and beauticians, the Walker Special Outfit was a convenient kit that included all the products necessary to employ the system. The outfit included six items: a handmade steel hot comb, a bristle hand brush, a ladies' scalp comb, Wonderful Hair Grower, Vegetable Shampoo, and Glossine. The fact that Walker is so often credited with (sometimes accused of) inventing the straightening comb speaks to the true saturation of the market the Walker system enjoyed. The numbers tell a similar story. In 1920, one year after Madam's death,

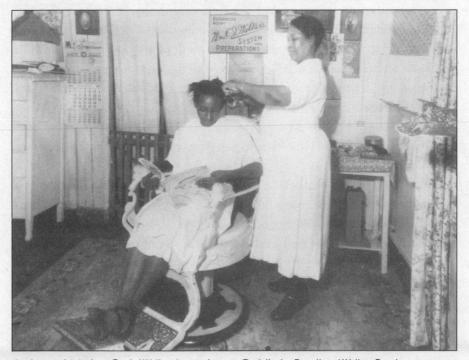

Authorized Madam C. J. Walker hair culturist. © A'Lelia Bundles, Walker Family Collection, Alexandria, Virginia.

the Walker company sales, including profits earned in Central America, South America, and the Caribbean, peaked at $595,000.

Following in the footsteps of the antebellum barbers of the past century, Walker, Malone, and other hair-care capitalists of the day invested a lot of money in the Black community. Walker, for instance, gave thousands of dollars to the National Association of Colored Women, the NAACP, the YWCA, the Tuskegee Institute, and many other Black social and civic organizations. She was very active in politics, championing the antilynching movement and women's rights. "My business is largely supported by my own people, so why shouldn't I spend my money so that it will go back into colored homes," Walker told a reporter in 1916 about her philanthropic efforts. Upon her death Walker made provisions to give away two-thirds of her net income. Annie Malone gave so much of her money away (one reason her business suffered in later years) that she was labeled a "freak giver." For example, over a ten-year period she gave more than twenty-five thousand dollars to Howard University's Medical School Endowment. Setting a precedent for the future of the hair-care industry, both Walker and Malone connected the progress of the race with the selling of their hair-care products. "To promote sales," writes Kathy Peiss in the *Harvard College Business History Review*, Malone and Walker "blurred the lines between business, philanthropy, community building and politics. Production and consumption were interwoven with ideologies of economic nationalism, racial advancement and female emancipation." When you bought a jar of Wonderful Hair Grower, in essence, you were investing in the future of the Negro race.

Both Malone and Walker have been compared to religious leaders, so compelling was their message and so zealous were their adherents. "I am not merely satisfied in making money for myself, for I am endeavoring to provide employment for hundreds of the women of my race," Walker announced to the audience of the National Negro Business League convention in 1914. "I had little or no opportunity when I started out in life, having been left an orphan. . . . I had to make my own living and my own opportunity! But I made it! That is why I want to say to every Negro woman present, don't sit down and wait for the opportunities to come. . . . Get up and make them!" All across the country women took Walker's message to heart, hit the pavement, and started selling hair-care preparations, often to the dismay of men who did not subscribe to the notion of females working outside the home. One Walker sales agent from Columbus, Ohio, sent the following letter to the company: "We have been able to purchase a home and overmeet our obligations. Before I started out as an agent in Madam Walker's employ, I made the regular working woman's wage, but at this writing I average $23 a week." Another grateful Walker agent from Florida wrote, "I have all I can do at home and don't have to go out and work for White people in kitchens and factories."

Although there is much dispute over who was the more financially successful of the two hair-care capitalists, it goes without saying that Madam C. J. Walker enjoys greater recognition in the annals of Black hair history. Bundles suggests several theories for the disparity. "Annie Malone had a much more reticent personality than Madam Walker [whereas] Madam had the ability to draw people to her," Bundles says. It wasn't just the personality, though, Walker's biographer hastens to add. "Madam was a great salesperson, she had great ideas, and she surrounded herself with talented people. Annie Malone had the misfortune of marrying a guy who basically sabotaged her business and sabotaged her." Bundles is referring to Malone's third husband, Aaron Malone, who attempted to wrest control of the business away from her shortly after the two were married. (Six years later, they were divorced.) "Madam Walker didn't have that same baggage," says Bundles. To seal their respective fates in hair history, Madam Walker died in 1919 at the height of her commercial success, while Malone died in 1957 after a series of scandals involving public lawsuits, bankruptcy, and accusations of tax fraud. Today the Walker family has made every effort to keep Madam Walker's memory alive. Their lobbying of the U.S. Postal Service resulted in the issuance of the first Madam C. J. Walker commemorative stamp in 1998. Annie Malone's relatives have not been as active in championing a posthumous memorial for Malone. Even in death, Malone's star remains in the shadows of Madam C. J. Walker.

Patterning themselves after Malone and Walker, several other Black-owned manufacturers became established in the early part of the century. Apex (founded by Sarah Spencer Washington, another great female hair-care pioneer), Kashmir Chemical Company, Rose Chemical Company, and Hair Care–Vim Chemical Company were all successful Black-owned companies that catered to the Black consumer, employed Black workers, and gave back to the Black community—a trend that would continue throughout modern times. As a group, women too enjoyed significant economic bene-fits in the early years of the twentieth century by selling hair-care prepara-tions or opening beauty salons. Throughout the South, some White people felt that because so many Black women were able to find employment in the hair-care industry, the supply of "rural and domestic labor" was being severely depleted. Lawmakers in Georgia were so distressed that they im-posed special punitive taxes on hairdressing establishments in an effort to destroy their businesses. In the northern cities, women and men were opening barbershops and hair salons so quickly that the trend was noted in *The New York Times* in 1917. There were so many hair-care establishments in Harlem, a reporter noted, that a stranger "gets the idea that members of the colored race must be afflicted with baldness, or think that their hair needs some sort of treatment." By 1920 in Chicago, the *Blue Book*, a direc-tory of Black businesses in the city, listed 211 barbers and 108 beauty sa-lons, numbers that did not include part-time or at-home establishments. The only other Black-owned businesses with similar numbers were gro-cery stores and delicatessens.

When the Great Depression hit, the boom years of the nascent Black hair-care industry came to a grinding halt. It was the beginning of the end for many Black-owned businesses like Poro Products. Walker Manufactur-ing, which had once enjoyed half-million-dollar annual sales, grossed a mere thirty-one thousand dollars in 1931. The company did not throw in the towel, but it did change its advertising and marketing strategy. A Depression-era advertisement for Walker's Tetter Salve and Tan-Off, for example, emphasized the Walker company's employment history with the "Race" and suggested that "in these times when we are so greatly con-cerned about jobs," a colored person could always earn money by selling Walker products. Tetter Salve and Tan-Off received only a brief mention in the entire full-page advertisement.

By the mid-1940s White manufacturers, having witnessed the profits and successes of the Black hair-care industry in the previous decades, were poised to enter this lucrative market. Taking advantage of the weakened state of Black businesses at the time, White-owned companies established themselves as key players in the hair game. There wasn't one clear indus-try leader, but together White-owned manufacturers like Vaseline and Dixie Peach held over 50 percent of the market share. The Poro Company held a mere 2.1 percent at this time, and Walker Manufacturing held on with a paltry 1.1 percent.

Although the Black-owned companies were hard hit by the Depression, World War II provided a welcome financial uplift for barbers, beauticians, and independent salespeople. At the 1946 National Beauty Culture League convention—a gathering of Black female hair-care professionals—it was reported that the war years drummed up four hundred million dollars in gross profits.

After the war, with competition from larger White manufacturers closing in, Black-owned hair-care companies focused on developing new products to stay one step ahead. Even though sales of pomades and pressing oils were vigorous during these years, the ultimate goal in the industry was to create a product that would straighten kinky hair "permanently." The ever-present hot comb worked fine, but the results only lasted until the hair met up with moisture—rain, humidity, or sweat. The first company to invent such a product would have millions of Black people (not to mention some Jewish and Italian people who found themselves blessed with kinky manes) clamoring to buy it. In 1948 the problem appeared to be solved. *Ebony* magazine rushed to print the story in its June issue, announcing "New Hair Culture Discovery: Mexican chemist claims process to make Negro hair straight, silky." Jose Calva, a Minneapolis-based chemical engineer famous for discovering a method to convert sheep's wool into minklike fur, used a similar process to create a product called Lustrasilk Permanent. This miracle cure for kinks was supposed to "give curly, uncombable, felty hair a silken, straight quality for months." The foamy Lustrasilk solution was to be sold only to licensed beauticians and came with a special electric comb and shampoo "capable of removing accumulations of pressing oil and other foreign matter impregnated in the hair."

Walker Manufacturing soon followed Dr. Calva's lead by announcing its own new long-lasting straightening solution. Less than a year after the debut of Lustrasilk Permanent, Walker introduced Satin Tress, promising a revolution in the industry. Satin Tress was advertised as a moisture-proof hair-conditioning treatment that would change the texture of hair after multiple applications. Like Lustrasilk, it was supposed to be applied by a professional beautician and included a special shampoo, the concoction itself, and a finishing conditioning cream. After a Satin Tress treatment, women still had to use a hot comb to straighten their hair, but it was supposed to take less time, less heat, and stay straight longer. As it said in the Satin Tress ads, this product will "rapidly and certainly retard your hair's stubborn tendency to 'go back.'" One year later, there was yet another alternative for achieving permanently straight hair. In 1950 Christina Jenkins, a housewife in Malvern, Ohio, invented and then patented the hair weave.

Chemical Creations: 1954–1979

Still, the real revolution in the industry did not occur until 1954, when a twenty-six-year-old Black upstart named George E. Johnson introduced a safe, "permanent" straightening system that could be purchased at retail and applied in the home. Ultra Wave Hair Culture was an invention of Johnson's, created in his off-hours as head production chemist for Fuller Products in Chicago, one of the most successful Black-owned businesses in twentieth-century America. While on the job, Johnson was approached by Orvile Nelson, a Black celebrity hairstylist who wanted to find a way to improve the crude potato starch and lye conks that he was using to straighten the hair of his well-known male clients, including Nat King Cole. When Johnson perfected the formula (basically mixing lye with petroleum instead of potatoes), he knew he was sitting on a veritable gold mine. Using a $250 loan, he started selling his Ultra Wave hair relaxer for men as the first item under his new company name, Johnson Products.

Just like Madam Walker before him, Johnson met with almost immediate success, not only because his product satisfied a need among Black consumers but because of his flair for business and marketing to the Black community. "It was a heck of a concept and George came along at the right time," Nelson told the *Chicago Tribune* in 1993. "He took it and made it dance in the street." Moreover, after years of White control of the industry, Johnson was a Black man making a product for Black people. Black consumers were delighted and supported Johnson Products wholeheartedly. By 1964 the company had recorded one million dollars in revenues, due in large part to the introduction of the women's relaxer, Ultra Sheen. Taking a cue from his predecessors, Johnson funneled much of his profits right back into the Black community by donating hundreds of thousands of dollars to various charities, setting up scholarships, and even funding a breakfast program for needy children on Chicago's impoverished South Side.

As Johnson continued to reap unprecedented success in the market, more White-owned health and beauty manufacturers became aware of the profitability of the Black hair-care market. Industry giants like Revlon and Clairol entered the market by acquiring smaller Black-owned companies that knew the products Black consumers desired. Revlon, for example, made its foray into Black hair care by purchasing a smaller company called Deluxol, whose key brand was Creme of Nature, a top-selling line of shampoos and conditioners. Until this time, the Black consumer had been routinely overlooked by the major White hair-care and beauty manufacturers. They were slow to respond to the needs of Black customers and rarely attempted to create special products to be marketed specifically to them. Some beauty care companies even went on record claiming the Black consumer market wasn't a profitable investment. Not surprisingly, throughout the 1960s, with consumer opinion firmly on their side, Johnson Products prevailed as the industry leader, holding 80 percent of the ethnic hair market for the majority of the decade.

When the rebelliousness of the late sixties and seventies hit the hair world, a lot of people were caught unaware. The popularity of the Afro and the other back-to-natural hairstyles had a lot of Black hairstylists running scared and angry. The "Black is beautiful" rhetoric caused a segment of consumers to renounce chemical products, hair straighteners, and "conformist" hairstyles. Black barbers and beauticians who watched their client base shrink as the Afro grew were forced to find innovative ways to stay solvent. "The Afro ran a whole generation of barbers out of business, put them on the unemployment lines," recalled East Cleveland barber Art McKoy, owner of the Super Fly barbershop. Nathaniel Mathis, a Washington, D.C.–based barber and beautician, kept himself afloat by proclaiming himself a first-class Afro expert. After watching several of his colleagues go out of business, Mathis went on a local television station to prove he could give anybody a big ol' Afro. His model was a blond housewife with straight hair. On camera Mathis proceeded to perm the White woman's hair, blow it out, cut it, and shape it until she had a really large bush. After that publicity stunt, Mathis was forever known as the Bush Doctor. Many Black stylists followed Mathis's lead, providing services like blow outs and precision trims to Afro wearers and creating ways to perm straight hair into an Afro style.

Hair-care manufacturers were equally concerned as retail sales of chemical relaxers and other straightening products dropped considerably. Some companies, in an effort to sabotage the Afro's staying power, went so far as to produce advertisements suggesting that natural styles were more damaging to the hair than chemical relaxers. Some companies, like the White-owned Clairol, attempted to use Black vernacular and the "Black is Beautiful" spirit to sell their products. "Free your 'Fro" is how Clairol pushed its oil sheens and sprays. Johnson Products Company, however, was left unscathed by the advent of the Afro. The politically charged coiffure actually added to the company's profitability. Instead of pushing his Ultra Wave and Ultra Sheen relaxers (which still accounted for about 50 percent of sales) to the revolutionary Blacks of the "movement," Johnson developed a line of moisturizing products made especially for natural hairstyles. In a relatively short amount of time, the average Black home in America was not complete without a jar of Johnson's blue hair grease. In keeping with the Afrocentric spirit of the movement, Johnson's Afro Sheen products were marketed with a tag line in Swahili: "Watu-Wazuri (Beautiful People) use Afro Sheen." The ubiquitous black-bottled products kept Johnson sitting pretty throughout the early seventies. In 1971 the company became the first Black-owned company to trade on the American Stock Exchange. That same year Johnson Products became the corporate sponsor of the TV dance show *Soul Train*, marking the first time a Black advertiser sponsored a nationally syndicated television show.

Johnson Products wasn't the only Black-owned business to make it big in this period. Between the late 1950s and the 1970s, several Black men and women started what would become multimillion-dollar companies by banking on the new hairstyles of the day. Edward Gardner, a former elementary school principal in Chicago, started Soft Sheen Products in 1964 with his wife, Bettiann, hawking homemade hair-care products out of the back of their car. In 1973 two former pharmacists in Atlanta, Cornell

McBride and Therman McKenzie, started experimenting with glycerin to create a product to make natural hair softer and more supple. Using themselves as guinea pigs, they finally perfected an oil-sheen spray and called it Sta-Soft Fro. The two friends mixed their product in the bathtub, bottled it themselves using homemade labels, and hit the road. By 1977 Sta-Soft had caught the attention of Chattem Drug and Chemical, makers of Nadinola skin (aka bleaching) cream. Chattem sent one of its Black employees, product manager Ed Rutland, down to Georgia to see if McKenzie and McBride wanted to discuss working together with Chattem. Instead Rutland, realizing the young company's potential, offered to buy them out for several hundred thousand dollars on the spot. The two bathtub chemists refused Rutland's offer, saying they were going to turn their company into a million-dollar enterprise on their own. Less than three years later, M&M Products posted sales of four million dollars, and the two founders hired Ed Rutland as their first director of marketing. Five years later, company sales were up to forty-three million dollars.

The Black hair-care industry was shaken in 1975 when the federal government instigated what appeared to be a racist conspiracy. That year the Federal Trade Commission ordered Johnson Products to add a warning label on its Ultra Sheen relaxer because the product contained lye (as did all relaxers at the time). George Johnson agreed to the label with the assumption that the same warning would be applied to all hair relaxers. But for unknown reasons the FTC did not force Revlon, Johnson's main competitor, to affix the label to its relaxer until twenty-two months later. During that almost two-year period, Revlon used the warning on Ultra Sheen to promote its relaxer as a "better and safer product." Although Revlon eventually had to affix a warning label, albeit one that was milder than Ultra Sheen's, the damage had been done to Ultra Sheen's reputation. Johnson eventually sued the FTC for the unfair treatment and won. "But Revlon was able to get their toehold in the Black hair market," says Rutland. Johnson told a reporter for the *Chicago Tribune* that the FTC incident almost destroyed the relaxer division of his business. "It was an absolute assassination of the brand name Ultra Sheen," Johnson railed. "The beneficiary here was Revlon." Though still posting multimillion-dollar sales, Johnson Products never rallied back to its position of industry Goliath after the FTC incident. The FTC has never gone on record with an explanation of this seemingly unfair behavior. By the end of the 1970s, Johnson's grip on the Black hair-care industry had sufficiently loosened to let other companies vie for the top spot. Edward Gardner's Soft Sheen was ready and waiting.

The Big Wet Eighties

On the streets people were calling it a Jheri Curl. Jheri Redding, a White Illinois farm boy turned hair-care entrepreneur, had invented a chemical process that converted straight (i.e., Caucasian) hair into curly hair. But Redding's invention wasn't intended to be used on kinky Black hair, and most hair-care manufacturers assumed that was the end of the story. Conventional wisdom said that tight, kinky hair could not be converted into loosely curled hair. One man, a self-taught inventor living in Southern California, thought otherwise. Willie Lee Morrow, author of several books on Black hair and the man who first mass-produced the plastic Afro pick in this country, had been tinkering with a chemical process to turn kinky hair curly since 1966. His wonder product did not make much of a splash until 1977, when he changed its name from the Tomorrow Curl to the California Curl, and traveled across the country demonstrating its versatility and ease. The California Curl, sold initially only to stylists, was widely accepted by the Black community and helped edge out the natural styles of the previous decade. "It is my belief that the acceptance and instant popularity of the 'California Curl' is that at long last Black brothers and sisters were provided with a hairstyle that was recognized as being significantly Black and provided an easily accomplished and simply maintained hair-do," Morrow wrote in his book *400 Years Without a Comb*. Soon Black- and White-owned manufacturing companies were rushing to create their own version of the California Curl for Black customers, excited by the potential profits of this product-heavy style. Even Jheri Redding (who would go on to build the still-thriving Nexxus empire), with the help of a Black colleague, reformulated his original product to adapt to Black hair. Coincidentally, Jheri Curl became the popular or layman's term to refer to all curly perms, much as Xerox is to copy machines. Willie Morrow responded in his book: "I feel no animosity because my idea was copied and exploited by the very same companies which had declined to do the research and development of a much needed product. Instead, I am gratified that I was able to introduce a process that has been accepted universally."

Edward Gardner's company took the lead in the Black hair-care market in 1979 with the introduction of the Care Free Curl relaxer, Soft Sheen's version of the curly perm. The Care Free Curl was applied in the salon at a cost of eighty to a hundred dollars, then maintained on a daily basis with an arsenal of moisturizers and curl activators. Consumers could expect to spend approximately five hundred dollars a year on Soft Sheen's maintenance products alone. The chemicals used in most Curl processes left the hair severely dehydrated, thus the constant need for lubricating oils, creams, and sprays. Gardner's Care Free Curl and various similar products like Pro-Line's Curly Kit (the first retail Curl product) were a manufacturer's dream because the style required both salon visits and maintenance products and was worn by men, women, and children. The Curl "was a gold mine for manufacturers," said Ed Rutland. The slick style spurred unprecedented industry growth, and not just for manufacturers of Curls but for companies who concentrated on making moisturizing products for Curl wearers. "The Jheri Curl is why Sta-Soft Fro got so far ahead," Rutland explained. "You needed a lot of glycerin to keep that Curl wet. As the Curl grew, Sta-Soft grew." Interestingly, Johnson Products was one of the

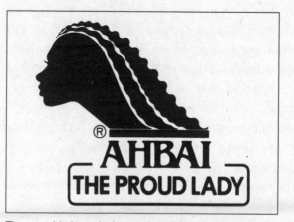

The proud lady symbol reminds consumers to buy Black!
Courtesy of the American Health and Beauty Aids
Institute.

few major manufacturers that did not get carried away with the Curl. While the rest of Black America was reveling in their juicy new hairdos, George Johnson tried rather unsuccessfully to diversify into the nonethnic (read White) and international hair-care markets. It was the beginning of the end for Johnson Products.

The eighties proved to be a significant decade in the hair-care industry. By 1980 Johnson Products had dropped from holding a 60 percent market share to 40 percent. Black-owned firms enjoyed continuous growth, owing much to the tremendous popularity of the Curl, but large White-owned companies were gaining momentum. Revlon at this time coincidentally started packaging its products in yellow and red bottles that looked almost identical to Soft Sheen's Care Free Curl line. In 1981, to protect themselves against White encroachment, ten Black hair-care manufacturers joined forces and founded the American Health and Beauty Aids Institute (AH-BAI). George Johnson was the founding chairman. Conceived as a resource and advocate for Black-owned businesses, the AHBAI's inaugural mission was to launch a three-million-dollar advertising campaign urging consumers to "buy Black." The founding members of the AHBAI commissioned Chicago-based artist Richmond Jones to design a silhouette of a Black woman—"the proud lady"—as their symbol. Members of the newly formed organization displayed "the lady" on all their products so customers could make informed choices at the checkout counter. For a time Black magazines like *Ebony, Essence,* and *Jet* supported the AHBAI's efforts by refusing to feature ads for Revlon products. Many White-owned companies were incensed by such tactics, claiming that AHBAI members were turning shampoo and conditioner into a racial issue rather than a simple question of hygiene. Both Revlon and Alberto Culver (makers of the TCB product lines) responded to the AHBAI's actions by using well-known Black entertainers in their advertisements.

As the current executive director of the AHBAI and the de facto industry spokesperson, Geri Duncan Jones spends a lot of time explaining exactly why this industry makes no bones about playing the race card. "These [Black-owned] companies not only manufacture products, [they] have actually established businesses where they are able to make a contribution—in the form of jobs, in the form of scholarships, in the form of assisting with voter registration—to the communities in which they serve," Jones says with passion. "Most of the companies that are not African-American owned are not even based in cities or areas where they employ a number of African-Americans, and if they do, they're not in management levels or there are few in management level positions." In the mid-1980s, companies like Revlon and Alberto Culver made overtures to the Black community by making charitable donations to Black organizations like the United Negro College Fund and the Jackie Robinson Foundation. But it was difficult for Black industry insiders to view these gifts as anything more than symbolic. A real commitment came from African-American businessman Commer Cottrell, then CEO of Pro-Line Corporation, who spent $3.5 million in 1990 to save two historically Black colleges from closing. "These are the kinds of contributions we're talking about," says Duncan Jones. "It's not superficial, it's real, and it makes a difference."

The struggle for market control was on in earnest by the time the president of Revlon's professional products division, Irving Bottner, made his infamous 1987 statement in *Newsweek* that led to the mock funeral protests. Throughout the industry, Black and White manufacturers were fighting for control of the billion-dollar industry. By 1988 White manufacturers dominated more than 50 percent of the market. As Bottner intimated, however, Revlon, Alberto Culver, Helene Curtis, and other like-minded White behemoths were not content with majority control; they wanted to dominate the industry. If this were any other industry, say, production of cheese or satellite dishes, one would expect healthy competition, but nothing is ever quite that simple when it comes the business of Black hair. "In order for us to survive in this world, economic stability is very important," says Jones thoughtfully. "The mom-and-pop restaurants are basically all gone. The funeral business is no longer just in our hands. The ethnic hair-care industry is one of the few industries where African-Americans still have a foothold. We don't want to see this go away also."

By the end of the eighties and into the early nineties, the ethnic hair-care industry had not slipped away from Black ownership completely, but it had witnessed some very significant changes. George Johnson and Joan, his wife of thirty-eight years, terminated their marriage, and as part of the divorce settlement George Johnson relinquished ownership of the company to his wife. In 1993 Joan sold Johnson Products to the White-owned

Ivax Corporation for a reported sixty-seven million dollars. Geri Duncan Jones's fears looked as if they might come to pass. Meanwhile the robust growth in the industry stemming from the wildly popular curly perms came to a messy end when people decided that the cost of replacing lubricant-stained pillowcases, shirt collars, and furniture wasn't worth a cute new hairdo. Though there was still a loyal core of Jheri Curl enthusiasts (many of them opting for the slightly less drippy S-Curl and the so-called dry curl, Wave Nouveau), the trend was over, soon to be replaced by more Afrocentric styles like braids, Afros, and cornrows. Market watchers like Ed Rutland, now executive vice president at a Manhattan public relations agency, says the industry hasn't been able to rally since the boom years of the Jheri Curl. "When the Curl went away, the market collapsed," Rutland reports forlornly. With hair-care trends emphasizing more natural styles, manufacturers were forced to focus on producing inexpensive maintenance products like conditioners and moisturizers while they prayed for a chemical comeback to spur growth.

Getting Back to Nature

At the end of the 1990 calendar year, *Essence* magazine, a benchmark of Black culture in the United States, urged its readers to embrace their African heritage with headlines like "Reclaiming Our Culture." The African-American moniker was not supposed to be just a name but a way of life. From holiday celebrations to family planning, living a more Afrocentric life was prescribed in order to travel the "path toward self-determination." Suddenly kente cloth patterns and Nigerian Barbie dolls were all the rage. Black women started wearing their hair in intricate African-inspired braided styles, which launched an enormously successful business for immigrant African hair braiders.

Hair-care manufacturers jumped right on the bandwagon. Black- and White-owned companies fell all over themselves trying to out-Africanize one another with new or improved product releases. Revlon introduced new lines of sprays and sheens named after African cultural groups, like Masai Polishing Mist and Fanti Moisturizing Hairdress. Alberto Culver's TCB line of products was now called TCB Naturals and was infused with exotic oils and herbs from Africa. Black-owned Bronner Brothers of Atlanta introduced an entire new product line under the name African Royale. Finally a relative newcomer to the scene decided the competition over the Motherland had to stop, so he set out to level the playing field.

In 1993 Brooklyn-based Shark Products was only two years old and already making million-dollar sales. The White-owned company manufactured mostly shampoos, conditioners, and variations of hair grease under the brand name African Pride. The products were packaged in the African nationalist colors of red, black, and green, the products contained ingredients that at one time supposedly grew in Africa, and the sweet scent of watermelon sprang from almost every package. Most consumers assumed that African Pride came from a Black manufacturer until company president Brian Marks decided to sue a smaller Black-owned company and his cover was blown. Shark sued three-month-old B&J Sales of Fayettville, Georgia, claiming that B&J, makers of the new African Natural product line, had violated trademark laws by using the word *African* in its product name. Having already successfully intimidated a different small Black-owned firm into changing its packaging, the Shark brass believed they owned the exclusive right to use the word *African* as well as the African nationalist colors. It was a ridiculous claim and one that seemed to validate the fear of many Black business owners that once White people entered the Black hair-care industry, they wouldn't rest until they put all Blacks out of business. After three months of grandstanding and threats, Shark dropped the lawsuit, and both companies continued to make African-inspired hair products in an uneasy truce. (As a footnote, Shark's African Pride was eventually bought by Revlon.)

The African Pride lawsuit was the culmination of every paranoia Black hair-care manufacturers felt about White encroachment in the Black hair business. Just one year later, consumers experienced their own nightmare. Had they only remembered the turn-of-the-century warnings to "be beautiful if you can, but don't burn your brains out in the process," a major disaster could have been avoided. Instead, in a quest for hair that moved, consumers got burned.

In 1994 the World Rio Corporation tried to pull off the ultimate get-rich-quick scheme, but it resulted in millions of dollars' worth of pain, suffering, and lawsuits instead of profits. The plan was to sell a miracle cure for kinky hair. (Sound familiar?) The product was called Rio and was marketed almost exclusively to Black American women. This wonder product was supposed to be an "all-natural chemical-free relaxer," created from flora and fauna found only in the Amazon rain forest. Sold exclusively through infomercials on late-night television, Rio was heralded as a breakthrough for Black women who craved hair that moved but were tired of using harsh chemical relaxers. "When you use chemicals, you go into bondage," a woman on the Rio infomercial intoned as she shook her flowing locs. "With Rio you are free." The woman on television made the process look so easy, so pleasant, invigorating even, with waterfalls splashing in the background.

In a few months, thousands of people had ordered their Brazilian miracle pack and waited for the herbs and spices to take root. Instead of straight, silky, bouncy hair, however, over two thousand Rio users experienced itchy scalps with oozing blisters, green hair, and/or complete hair loss. Only after a class-action lawsuit was lodged against the company was it was discovered that the Rio concoction was actually chock-full of highly acidic chemicals. The FDA closed the doors of the World Rio Corporation, and hordes of Black women went back to being chemical prisoners.

After Rio, African Pride, and over three hundred years of waiting for that perfect product to make Black hair straight, shiny, and long, it was high time for the weave industry to take off. While the weave process—adding synthetic or real hair to one's own tresses—had existed for conceivably thousands of years, the early 1990s saw Black women take to the add-on hair game like never before. Once an option for cancer victims and sufferers of alopecia, hair weaves became the ultimate accessory. Consequently, a once insignificant industry—human hair import—boomed. By the late nineties, 1.3 million pounds of human hair valued at $28.6 million were imported from countries like China, India, and Indonesia, where poor women sell their hair by the inch. Once the hair arrives in this country, already sterilized and styled, it goes on to wholesalers who sell the goods to beauty supply shops, beauty parlors, and hair retailers. Previously the domain of Jewish merchants, the human hair selling business in urban meccas from New York to Los Angeles is now dominated by Korean immigrants.

Building Bridges

At the dawn of the twenty-first century, the ethnic hair-care industry definitely looks different from when it started more than a hundred years ago. The manufacturing side of the industry is practically owned by large White-owned corporations like Cosmair and Alberto Culver. Johnson Products was sold again in 1998, to White-owned Carson Products. George Johnson tried to buy his company back but was beaten out by the Georgia-based company. The base of operations for Johnson Products is now in Savannah, Georgia, ending a Chicago hair-care affair. Soft Sheen Products was also sold in 1998 to French cosmetics giant L'Oreal. And most recently, Pro-Line Corporation was sold to Alberto Culver.

In a surprising twist that caught industry insiders unaware, the distribution of ethnic hair care products is primarily in the hands of Asian immigrants. "Right now Asian companies represent at least 45 to 50 percent of the total distribution of our hair-care products, which is a tremendous amount," Geri Duncan Jones declares incredulously. Other industry insiders place that number closer to 60 percent. "No one ever dreamed fifteen years ago that this would be the case today," says Duncan Jones.

The story of how Korean immigrants entered the Black hair-care market is an interesting one. Koreans entered the hair-import trade in America soon after the first wave of immigration in 1965, because they had established links with suppliers in Asia. With the links to the African-American customer being forged in urban markets by other Korean business owners, it was only a matter of time before some innovative minds would enter the retail and distribution end of the Black hair-care industry. While Black-owned mom-and-pop shops were going out of business in the Reagan-era eighties, Korean immigrants were banding together to form credit associations that would provide the start-up cash for new business ventures, effectively bypassing the bank loan process. Comparatively speaking, the cost of opening a Black hair-care supply shop was rather low, and a good jar of hair grease practically sold itself. The success of one store owner inspired another. When asked why he started selling hair-care products for Black people, Tong Park, owner of the massive Beauty Island retail shop in Milwaukee, Wisconsin, said he got the idea from his friends who own similar stores in Chicago. Park says he stays on top of trends and educates himself about different products by listening to his customers' requests, reading all the manufacturers' information, and meeting regularly with sales reps. "I don't care what color the people are," says Park matter-of-factly. "It's who has the money and who has the supply." Today, there's even a Korean-language trade magazine, *Beauty Times*, with an editorial content dedicated exclusively to the latest in Black hairstyles and trends.

The one aspect of the industry that Blacks continue to dominate is the barbering and salon business. Geri Duncan Jones attributes this success to the fact that Black people—men and women—feel more comfortable having their hair done by someone with Black hair. This being the case, Black salon owners are not waiting to lose this legacy as well and are starting to diversify their salons, offering services to Whites, Asians, and Latinos as well as Blacks.

Diversity is what Geri Duncan Jones is trying to preach to the manufacturing members of the AHBAI as well. Even though the industry has lost two of its greatest representatives, Johnson Products and Soft Sheen, Duncan Jones is unwilling to entertain the idea that the Black hair-care manufacturers will go the way of the mom-and-pop restaurants of the past. "I don't see this industry dying at all," Duncan Jones insists. "What I see now in our communities is a lot of smaller companies have sprung up, and these companies are more concerned with selling at fair prices and maintaining their business rather than trying to get huge volume and possibly putting themselves in a precarious position." These companies are also the ones that will continue to invest in the Black community with scholarships, jobs, and training opportunities. In order to be more than just a blip on the radar screen, however, Duncan Jones encourages AHBAI members to investigate making hair-care and cosmetic products for more than just the Black population.

That's what eco-friendly companies like Paul Mitchell and Aveda are doing as they inch into the Black hair-care market. John Paul DeJoria, CEO of Paul Mitchell, refuses to categorize his company in terms of White or Black. "We make hair products for textures of hair, not colors of skin," says DeJoria. "There are supposedly only four colors of skin—black, white, red, yellow—but there are hundreds of different textures of hair." DeJoria also actively funnels his profits into nonprofit organizations supporting the environment, AIDS research, and training for Black hairstylists. Even the advertisements for Paul Mitchell Products highlight diversity, often showcasing Black, White, and Asian models in the same ad. With an operating agenda like that, the us-against-them feelings of the past hardly seem relevant.

And the Winner Is . . .

On October 9, 1999, George Johnson and Edward Gardner mingled in the ballroom of Chicago's stately DuSable Museum of African American History, along with nearly four hundred other people. Almost everyone in attendance was a celebrity in the hair-care industry, including stylists, corporate manufacturers, and a few relatives of Madam C. J. Walker. This cadre of distinguished guests was on hand to celebrate the AHBAI's first ever Hall of Fame Industry Awards, billed as "the Emmy of the ethnic hair-care industry." Many of the revelers were also nominees for one of the evening's twenty-two awards. George Johnson's Johnson Products and Edward Gardner's Soft Sheen Products were both up for Company that Revolutionized the Industry. Revlon also sent a representative to the event because it too had been nominated. Madam C. J. Walker was receiving recognition for revolutionizing the industry, as was Annie Turnbo Malone. Though expectations were high, tension was remarkably low. "It was probably the first event that we ever had where everyone came together and there wasn't any concern or fear or hostility or any of that," says Geri Duncan Jones, who helped organize the black-tie extravaganza. There was a newfound sense of camaraderie among the major players in the industry— Black, White, and Asian—that was palpable throughout the evening's activities. Soft Sheen was declared the Company that Revolutionized the Industry, and Care Free Curl was deemed the Brand that Revolutionized the Industry. "At this point there are no enemies," says Jones. "We recognize that it is a free enterprise system, and there are other companies out there that are manufacturing these products, and it doesn't look like they're going anywhere anytime soon. We've just kind of learned to work with them."

A Life in Hair:
Erye Anderson, Octogenarian

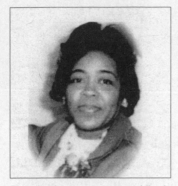

Erye Anderson, courtesy of Freda Mayes.

I was working for General Motors, and the job market was getting bad because of the recession in 1953. I thought I might have to be laid off. I went into the hair business because I knew it was good business. With our people we always have to do our hair.

I went to Lydia's School of Beauty Culture in Chicago. I would go to school at night from 6 P.M. to 8 P.M. and I'd have to stay late on Fridays. We had to learn about the history of the hair and the skin and about the anatomy of the hair. During my time at school, I had the highest grades in my class, and when I finished they told me I had the highest grades of any student, day or night. When you graduated, you had to take an exam downtown for your license. Usually it takes two days to take the exam, but because of my high average, they said I could do it in one day. Within a week or two, I had my license in Springfield and haven't given it up since.

I got my license in 1954. Within six months I had more customers than I knew what to do with. They weren't giving Black people perms then. We were more or less steaming it. I *was* giving perms to White people even though I didn't want to. I had a few White customers from Lincolnwood, and they said I did their hair better than anybody else. For Black people I did shampooing, pressing, conditioning, and styling, of course. The pompadours and pageboys were really popular.

I had a little salon built in the house in the basement. I did hair every day. I'd get home from GM at about 4:42 P.M. and then work until 12 A.M. some nights. The Afro didn't do a thing to my business. Everybody wanted their hair straight. Of course my husband wore an Afro, and he was a handsome fellow, but his family looked at him and said, "Oh, Delmo, you've gone and made your hair nappy."

Now the Jheri Curl was good for me. I used to make seventy-five dollars a head, and I could do four heads a day. It was a big turnaround for my economy. I made more money doing Jheri Curls than I was making at GM. But you have to be careful in this business. People have been known to get tuberculosis from inhaling all the smoke and chemicals, and Jheri Curls were really dangerous because they had a lot of ammonia.

There's something about beauty culture that gets in your bloodstream. And if you like it, it's hard to give up. It did pay off quite nicely for us. We prospered quite a bit. You can really do well in the hair business.

I did hair for about forty-one years, but I finally had to quit three years ago. People tell me, "Oh, Ms. Anderson, when are you going to start doing hair again?" and I have to say, "Ms. Anderson is out of business forever."

5

Politically Incorrect: Black Hair's New Attitude, 1980–1994

"What Farrah Fawcett did for the cascading mane, Bo Derek is doing for braids," *Newsweek* magazine proclaimed in 1980.

Ironically, the era that began with Blacks exploring a new visual aesthetic of natural, nappy hair and African-inspired styles ended with a White woman being championed by the mainstream as the embodiment of beauty for wearing one such look. In 1979 Bo Derek made the movie *10*. In it she wore her hair in cornrows with beads on the end, the same style that Cicely Tyson had worn more than a decade earlier. By 1980, on the pages of *Time* and *Newsweek* and in the lexicon of the population at large, cornrows had come to be known as "Bo Braids." Even those mainstream publications that took the time to note the African roots of the style seldom included photos of Black women wearing them.

Some liked to point to Bo Derek as an example of America's embracing a multicultural, more inclusive beauty ideal. The response was not favorable on all fronts, however. The African-American community and Black women in particular saw it as adding insult to injury. "I saw danger in Bo Derek," remembers *Ms.* magazine's former editor in chief, Marcia Gillespie. "What offended me was that it was bad enough that they were going to tell me that she was the most beautiful woman in the world, but then to put her in cornrows as if to cover all of the bases." After years of being seen as the anti-beauty, Black women now had to face something that was essentially stripped of its historical legacy and given acclaim only after being adopted by a White, blond woman. In an interview shortly after *10*'s release, Roberta Flack, who had been wearing her natural hair braided for some time, expressed her anger. "Black women were wearing cornrows long before Bo Derek," she told *The Christian Science Monitor*. "I took issue that [Whites] made such a big thing about Bo Derek and cornrows. I can see this Bo Derek doll going out, the '10' doll, with braids. And they [Whites] will make a zillion dollars off of it." In a *Jet* magazine article headlined "On Scale of 1 to 10, Blacks Rate 'Angry' Over Bo Derek's Hairdo Fad," stylists, celebrities, and other Black women and men echoed Flack's sentiments. Blacks overwhelmingly felt as though a cultural legacy had been literally whitewashed.

Bo Braids were indeed sweeping the White hair-care industry. The style was expensive, generally between one hundred and three hundred dollars, could take from four to fourteen hours to complete, and often needed to be redone within a week. Yet White women were flocing to places like Le Braids Cherie, a braids-only salon that opened in Hollywood, for the new look. New York City's Pierre Mitchell Salon charged five hundred dollars to braid White women's hair and add accessories like semiprecious stones. Women with short hair got extensions, and those with thin hair had to get it crimped so the plaits would stay in. New York women looking to spend less could go to a beauty salon connected to the YWCA in Harlem, a shop that had been doing cornrows since the mid-sixties. And the style was not only popular in the trend meccas of LA and New York; even White teens and adults in places like suburban Detroit were scrambling for it.

Although she was largely silent on the subject at the time, Bo Derek was always aware of the origins of the style that made her so famous. She and her husband, John Derek, used to do their grocery shopping in an African-American neighborhood in Southern California, where John would often see cornrowed styles that he thought would look good on his young wife. When Bo landed the ten-minute role as the object of Dudley Moore's obsession in *10*, John Derek was determined to get full mileage out of her screen time. With the permission of director Blake Edwards, Bo had her hair braided and history was made.

Bo Derek was not the first White person to adopt a traditionally Black look. There had been hints of White interest in the Afro and other Black hairstyles as early as the sixties. Hippies had been braiding and cornrowing their hair for years. In 1969 Washington, D.C., Afro specialist Nat "The Bush Doctor" Mathis had Afroed a White woman's hair for a live television audience. Art Garfunkel, Elliot Gould, Barbra Streisand, and *Welcome Back Kotter*'s Gabe Kaplan all wore the style. Afro wigs in a rainbow of colors were available in the pages of *Essence*, at stores such as Macy's, and as far away as Japan.

When taken in historical perspective, mainstream White adoption of these styles was groundbreaking. After centuries of African-Americans taking hair cues from Whites, in the seventies White Americans began to do the reverse. However, there were major differences. While White Americans were adopting some traditionally Black styles, the situation was only superficially comparable to what Blacks had been doing. A White woman with an Afro-like hairstyle or braids was "cool" and trendy. A Black woman with a straight bob hairstyle may have been trendy, but she was also more likely to get a job and to be deemed acceptable and more easily integrated into society. The White woman's aesthetic choices could hinge primarily on the look and very little on the sociopolitical or cultural relevance of its origins. And commodification and appropriation of these styles did not automatically translate into wholehearted acceptance and equality of African-centered looks. In her book *Unbearable Weight: Feminism, Western Culture, and the Body*, feminist philosopher Susan Bordo notes that in Bo Derek, and by extension all White women who wore cornrows, there was a privilege that was "so unimpeachably White as to permit an exotic touch of 'otherness' with no danger of racial contamination."

While Bo Braids were the most obvious and far-reaching example of the growing appropriation and depoliticization of Black hairstyles, they were only the beginning. In the 1980s Black hair—even when worn by White people—was about expressing one's individuality. If the Afro was meant to represent group pride and unity, the endless array of styles and variations that followed in its wake were to show individuality and uniqueness. In certain cases, Black hair still remained an issue of political and social contention in America, and some Blacks risked professional suicide over the styles they brought to the workplace. But as White women briefly flirted with cornrows and braids, the majority of Black women and men were moving on, reconnecting with straight hair, and trying new curly perms as well as experimental shapes, colors, and cuts. The time was a virtual visual free-for-all.

The eighties and the early years of the nineties were both a political and a visual anomaly in American history. While the ultraconservatism of the fifties could only be countered by the outrageousness of the anything-goes sixties and the further freewheeling look of the seventies, the eighties seemed to be without soul, connection, or purpose. Neon colors, mousse, Velcro, shoulder pads, and Spandex had no aesthetic predecessors. Black hair, instead of bucking the trends of mainstream America and continually reinventing itself in natural styles, ran en masse back to the no-lye relaxers. African-American women who had once stopped traffic with their gravity-defying 'fros were now as feathered, dyed, and silky smooth as their White peers. Hair was labeled "fun," and the eighties seemed determined to liberate follicles from any political or sociological weight. Black hair remained adornment, but now a chemically altered type.

Under Attack: Braids in the Workplace

While White women were getting braids for prices way below market value from Black women on the beaches of Caribbean islands or paying big bucks at expensive salons around the United States, Black women began making headlines of their own over braided styles. However, the reasons and their implications were altogether different.

In 1981 Renee Rogers, a ticket agent for American Airlines, was fired for wearing cornrows. She filed a discrimination suit that eventually went to the federal courts. Judge Abraham D. Sofaer of the Federal District Court of New York rejected her argument that the style evoked her African heritage, observing that she adopted the style shortly after the release of the film *10*. Following Rogers's case, African-American women continued to be reprimanded or dismissed from work over their decision to wear cornrows and braids. Other employers who prohibited braids in general or cornrows in particular included the Atlanta Urban League, Howard University Hospital, American Airlines (the director of corporate relations at the time said that braids were inconsistent with the airline's "businesslike, clean, fresh image"), and the Metropolitan Police Department in Washington, D.C.

In June 1987 a string of cases involving the issue began bringing national attention and even gaining the support of some unlikely allies. In 1987 Pamela Walker, a full-time teacher and doctoral student at the University of Illinois at Chicago, who worked part time at the Chicago Regency Hyatt, was fired when she arrived at work with cornrows. After Walker filed a complaint with the Equal Employment Opportunity Commission (EEOC) the hotel offered to reinstate her. Six months later, in January 1988, the Marriott Hotel in downtown Washington, D.C., sent home part-time employee Pamela Mitchell because of her "extreme, cornrowed hairstyle." The twenty-five-year-old, who filed a complaint with the District of Columbia's Office of Human Rights, gained national attention and even appeared on *CBS This Morning* to discuss her situation. On the show Mitchell said that her employer had a "discriminatory as well as a fashion problem." The case grabbed the attention of the media as well as the support of Jesse Jackson, then a candidate for the Democratic presidential nomination, and actress and former braid-wearer Bo Derek. The Marriott Hotel reviewed the case and welcomed Mitchell back to her position, having decided that her style was "acceptable." The hotel maintained, however, that even though Mitchell's hair was neat and unadorned, "other cases involving other kinds of cornrows might not be acceptable."

Two months later the nation's capital was the location of another braids case. Cheryl Tatum, thirty-seven, was a restaurant cashier at the Hyatt Regency Crystal City in suburban D.C. During Tatum's first two weeks at work she received compliments on her hair, which was styled in tight braids. Things changed when a supervisor told her to pull the braids into a bun to comply with the company's dress code. Tatum complied, but three weeks later the personnel director, Betty McDermott, told her to take out the braids, saying that the Hyatt prohibited "extreme and unusual hairstyles." According to Tatum, McDermott added, "I can't understand why you would want to wear your hair like that anyway." Tatum refused to change the style, calling her braids "an expression of my heritage, culture, and racial pride. They are impeccably groomed, carefully wrought, and cost-efficient." Furthermore, Tatum said that she wasn't interested in adopting a "White European style." Tatum was fired and promptly filed a suit with the EEOC. After the case gained national attention, John R. Hamilton, a hotel executive, issued a directive to the Hyatt Hotels saying that "well-groomed, neat, clean braided hair worn by females without any beads or jewelry is to be considered acceptable and not contrary to our image," but individual hotels were left free to determine if braids fit in with their location and clientele.

Following these cases and many others around the nation, the issue of braids and cornrows in the workplace became a political one. Janice Davis, a D.C. attorney, organized the Coalition for Cultural Equality to support women on the cornrows issue. Along with Jesse Jackson's Operation PUSH, the group organized boycotts of the Hyatt and focused national attention on the issue. Jackson threatened to boycott the Hyatt chain while on the campaign trail if the policy was not changed. Women's groups also lent their support to the cause. "It's outrageous that any person's job should depend on a hairstyle when the hairstyle has nothing to do with the ability to perform a job," said Molly Yard, then president of the National Organization for Women. The cornrow controversy was called a "workers' rights issue" by Ron Richardson, executive director of the Hotel and Restaurant Workers Union. Local 25 of this Washington, D.C., labor group held a petition drive to demand that the Hyatt and Marriott hotels end their hair discrimination practices. The petition sought reinstatement and financial compensation for all employees affected by the hairstyle policies, immediate revision of employee policies banning cornrows, and a public apology to the women.

The EEOC ruled that the Hyatt Hotels engaged in racial discrimination by prohibiting Black women from wearing their hair in cornrows. The commission allows employers to adopt any grooming standards they deem appropriate for the image they seek to project, as long as those standards are applied in a nondiscriminatory manner. Lawyers in the cornrow cases argued that by singling out braids, Black women were being disproportionately affected, which was therefore discriminatory. The EEOC ruling was cited in future court cases and federal and state discrimination claims as evidence that federal antibias laws protected cornrows as a distinct expression of Black cultural heritage.

Labor attorney Eric Steele, an attorney for many of the Washington-based women involved in the braid cases, estimated that over a thousand women had been victims of the bans on cornrows. He believed they all should be entitled to cash settlements under terms of the EEOC decision. He went so far as to liken the public stance taken by Cheryl Tatum and Pamela Mitchell to Rosa Parks's 1955 refusal to give up her seat on a Montgomery, Alabama, bus. "Employers will know across the country that they cannot engage in this kind of discrimination," he said at a press conference about the issue. "[Black women] will know they have a right to come forth and show part of their heritage without worrying about being disciplined or discharged by their employer."

While the majority of braids discrimination cases involved women who worked in the service or hospitality industry, braids were increasingly being worn by many African-American female professionals, including doctors, lawyers, teachers, clerical workers, flight attendants, and ministers. Women and their stylists reasoned that braids offered practical and healthful advantages, but employers argued that they did not fit the "corporate image." Many employers were intimidated by the statements they thought the braids made. In a *Wall Street Journal* article, Maury Hanigan wrote, "[Braids] may bring attention to the fact that the candidate comes from a different culture, with a different value system. . . . That strikes fear into the minds of hiring managers." In a 1988 *Essence* article on the subject, business-education teacher Yvonne M. Simmons, who is African-American, agreed that these styles were inappropriate. "You either look professional or you don't," she is quoted as saying. "I see very little difference between a punk cut, purple hair, dredlocs or braids. They are all extreme hairstyles that don't belong in the office."

Black women now had to contend with one more issue as they attempted to enter and move up the ladder in the workplace. Aside from the possible repercussions of racism and sexism, many now had to hope that their choice of hairstyle—hair that was not unnaturally colored, spiked, or mohawked—would not offend or scare their bosses. In 1988, Barbara A. Brown, acting associate dean of students at Spelman, Atlanta's all-female Black college, said that she told each student that "she has to decide what's more important:

the way that she wears her hair or the position she is currently seeking." Some women decided they did not want to work in environments they saw as hostile to their ethnic expressions. Image consultant Harriette Cole suggests to her clients that they decide what their professional goals are and "tailor your hair and style so that you stay on your path." She stresses that the standards of acceptable appearance vary from industry to industry and that if her clients are aware of the standard, they can then decide if an industry is one they want to work in. She warns that "if you choose to work on Wall Street, you have to figure out how you're going to be a part of it because Wall Street is not going to change for you." *Essence*, in the midst of the braids-in-the-workplace uproar, ran a pictorial on appropriate "9 to 5 Braids" to offer women practical, work-friendly styles, such as braided French rolls, topknots, and chignons.

In an interesting twist, a White woman underwent a similar experience in October 1991. LaCosta Resort Hotel and Spa in San Diego sent a woman home who wore braids to her job as a hostess. Kerry Powers had been a hostess at the restaurant for three years and had her hair braided with beads to diversify her look as a model. She was told to change the style or wear a wig because the style was too "eccentric." The hotel maintained that Powers was not fired but that hers was a case of "self-termination" for refusing to restyle her hair.

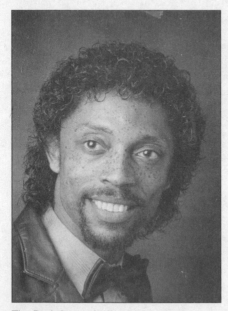

The Bush Doctor's Wave Noveau.
Courtesy of Nathaniel Mathis.

The Curly Perm: Its Heyday and Its Fall

Things on the hair front were not all dismal for Blacks in the post-Afro days. In fact, a new product gave many consumers a reason to celebrate. It was called the curly perm but had come to be more popularly known as the Jheri Curl. The Curl was the pinnacle of the intersection between a consumer market looking to explore new visual avenues and a beauty manufacturing industry looking to regain some of the ground it lost during the product-deficient Afro days. The style was heralded as a low-maintenance, versatile wake-up-and-go epiphany.

Grandmothers and kindergartners were as likely to be seen with a Curl as any other group. "Fresh. Hot. You ignite the day and blaze the night," read a Care Free Curl ad. "You're the new attitude." For those Black men who just couldn't bear to cut off their high-standing Afros, the Curl gave the option for a Lionel Richie wet look or a slicker curly ponytail. Short hair could be Curled to give the look of a close-cropped head of minicurls. Any women's style could be updated with a Curl. Bobs, wedge cuts, and Farrah Fawcett Feathers were all Curl-able. The promise of needing nothing more than activator (commonly referred to as "Jheri Curl Juice") and a shower cap (to keep in the moisture) in order to obtain a head of hair that was close to the desired "good" hair of the light-skinned Black elite of the past created a hair revolution.

Interestingly, the Curl phenomenon was not just about a way to look good but about a way to look good *economically*. A Care Free Curl print ad appearing just in time for the Christmas holidays targeted children with "It's easy to care for, light on the budget and kids love the different looks they can get. So let your kids ring in the season looking better than ever. . . ." April Garrett, a documentarian and writer from Baltimore, says she got a Curl as an adolescent because it was the cheapest way for her mother to take care of her hair. "My reasons for getting a Curl were more financial than anything else for my single mother."

Whites and Blacks who had finally adjusted to seeing big Afros, headwraps, cornrows, and the other natural styles that were worn in the seventies now had to contend with legions of Black men and women of all ages and complexions wearing not only Curls but in many cases see-through plastic shower caps out in public. The shower caps were worn to keep the Curls moisturized. While it was suggested that people only wear them overnight, many wanted to make sure that their style would be as wet and nourished as possible at all times and took to keeping the shower caps on more often than not. "I grew up in the eighties, and one of my biggest memories is of riding the public bus every morning to school with my mom and asking her why there were people with shower caps on their head," remembers writer Lauren Epps. "I was so confused. My mom would just tell me not to stare and that she'd explain when we got home."

Within months the curly perm was everywhere. Celebrities adopted it as readily as the general public. From New Edition to Debbie Allen to singer Nikolas Ashford (who called his a "lion's mane"), it was the look to have. Then in the early days of 1984, the world witnessed a tragedy that would have seemed more likely as a *Saturday Night Live* sketch but happened in real life and was replayed again and again on televisions around the world.

"Michael Jackson had been shot," read *Time* magazine's cover story. "That was the first reaction to those nearby when he grabbed the back of his head and screamed. It was not a bullet wound that made him scream, though it was almost as bad. Jackson's head was on fire."

On January 27, 1984, at approximately 6 P.M., one of the world's biggest stars, Michael Jackson, was shooting a commercial for the soft-drink giant Pepsi at Los Angeles' Shrine Auditorium. Jackson and his brothers, along with three thousand extras, were starting the fifth take of the day's filming. Standing at the top of a stairway, Jackson was to begin a dancing descent to the floor as fireworks exploded behind him. Halfway down he felt something on his head but thought it was just one of the stage lights, so he continued. He then felt a jolt of pain and cried out. Miko Brando, actor Marlon's son and a Jackson security aide, was the first to help, burning his own fingers while running them through Jackson's sizzling hair. The fire was extinguished within seconds. A nurse who happened to be in the audience, Shirley Morgan, wrapped ice in a T-shirt and immediately applied it to Jackson's head, a move doctors later said was instrumental in preventing major burning and scarring. Paramedics arrived on the scene and rushed the superstar to Cedars-Sinai Medical Center, where he made a full recovery.

Whenever something slightly out of the ordinary happens to the famous it is given press coverage. But Jackson's accident was front-page news the world over. The reason was not simply that the incident happened at the peak of his *Thriller* success but that the mishap was so *strange*. It was not normal for a head of hair to catch on fire, particularly if it was not near an open flame. However, in the history of humankind, it was also not normal for one head of hair to be as laden down with flammable products as Jackson's was.

Was it the activator? Was it the special effects? Accusations came from both sides. Cultural critic Kobena Mercer wrote that Michael Jackson's accident was interpreted by some as "punishment for the profane artificiality of his image." Daryoush Maze, an extra on the Pepsi set, told *The New York Times* that there was "just blue smoke from all the stuff he had in his hair." Friends of the singer told *Time* that his hair had no flammable pomade or hair spray on it, which seems unlikely. Jackson himself was reportedly irritated at the insinuations that his Curl had been partially to blame. A spokesperson for Jackson, John Branca, eventually conceded that the singer's hair *had* been treated with pomade for the commercial, but he believed a smoke-bomb canister may have exploded on Jackson's head. Others said that the fire was ignited by sparks from fireworks that were going off during the filming.

The media used the case to bemoan the growing lack of safety on Hollywood sets. But for the curly perm, it was a sign of bad things to come. By 1984 people were still wearing the Curl, but it was definitely losing its coolness. After Michael Jackson's accident, countless jokes were made about how Curl wearers better take special precautions because they might spontaneously combust.

The Black pop culture machine was also turning its back on the style. In Robert Townsend's 1987 film *Hollywood Shuffle*, a local thug was reduced to a sniveling wimp when his activator was taken away and his once slick hair matted and renapped before the audience's eyes. The parody illuminated a problem that most of Black America was already aware of: Curls were difficult to maintain, had a distinct and not altogether pleasant odor, and were messy. Countless pillowcases and chair backs were ruined with activator stains. The arsenal of products required for upkeep of the moisture-dependent style was expensive. More spoofs were to follow. They included Eddie Murphy's *Coming to America* and the family that made its fortune off its Curl company, Soul Glo, but left its true mark with telltale activator stains wherever they rested their heads. The popular early nineties Black sketch comedy

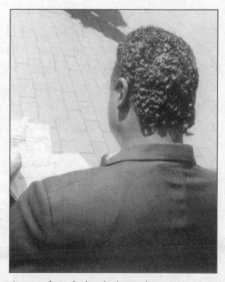

A view from behind: the curly perm.
© Alfonso Smith.

show *In Living Color* dedicated significant amounts of its early material to lampooning the Curl (the irony being that the show's creator, Keenan Ivory Wayans, had played the "juiceless" tough guy in *Hollywood Shuffle*).

Nevertheless, many Blacks hung on to their Curls for years to come. Atlanta engineer Vance Thomas, fifty-two, who got his first Curl in the early eighties, never let go because he believed that his own hair, which he prefers to keep long, was too difficult to comb. "It's more conducive to styling and controlling," Thomas explains. The division between the Curl-ers and the Curl-nots was the beginning of marked regional differences in African-American hair. Curly perms, on men and women, remained popular throughout the eighties and early nineties in the South and Midwest and on the West Coast. The North moved away from it, with women usually chemically straightening their hair and men wearing short, natural cuts.

Aside from having their cool passes revoked, Curl wearers were coming to be seen as being ashamed of their Blackness. In his essay "Black Hair/Style Politics," Kobena Mercer notes that after the Michael Jackson/Pepsi incident the Curl was read as both a bad imitation of White hair and representative of a "diseased state of Black consciousness." Ironically, most often those men and women who labeled Curl wearers as sellouts had no ideological problems with permed relaxers. It was as if only one culturally conscious chemical treatment was allowed by the Black Thought Police. In a scene from Spike Lee's 1987 film *School Daze*, two male characters have a "How Black are you?" confrontation. One ends the argument with the following: "Don't ever question whether I'm Black. In fact, I was gonna ask your country Bama ass why do you put those Jheri Curl drip-drip chemicals in your Black nappy hair?" The hairstyle that once swept a Black nation was now being represented in this seminal example of Black film as regressive and not culturally Black.

Men, Hip-Hop, and Eighties Hair

As Jheri Curls and Michael Jackson were taking the country by storm, there was another movement under way. Hip-hop culture was taking shape, spreading across the nation, and infiltrating mainstream America. Hip-hop—which included rap music, graffiti, break dancing, and deejaying—was a phenomenon that began in New York's South Bronx and was to have a major impact on the way young Black men and women styled themselves. For the first time since jazz debuted, a lifestyle anchored by music and created by Blacks melded creative musicality with the urgent messages of urban life. Historian and popular culture critic Tricia Rose wrote in her *Black Noise: Rap Music and Black Culture in Contemporary America*, "Hip hop style [forged] local identities for teenagers who understood their limited access to traditional avenues of social status attainment." The young men and women who were a part of the burgeoning hip-hop nation appropriated and redefined the music, dance, and styles of America and stamped them with their own unshakably cool, edgy trademark.

A style piece written for *The Washington Times* noted, "Nobody has ever accused Black men of lacking originality, or not having style. Right now, many of them are expressing their uniqueness through what they do with the curly/kinky/wavy/nappy stuff on their heads." There were many popular styles for young African-American men, but they all derived from the Philly fade, named so because of its origins in Philadelphia. Some men had worn a version of the look as early as the fifties, and by the eighties it was the keystone of Black male visual expression. The fade is short on the sides and in the back and gradually lengthens as it approaches the top of the head. Olympic track star Carl Lewis helped to popularize the look, and there was a constant give-and-take of styles among celebrities and young men. Malcolm-Jamal Warner, Theo on *The Cosby Show*, constantly changed his style, as did athletes and musicians. The hair on top could be worn several inches high, an extreme example being the high-top fade worn by rapper Kid of Kid 'N Play. There were the patent-leather waves (worn by actor Blair Underwood), the high-rise (a favorite of Arsenio Hall), and the Mike Tyson sideways part. Other variations on the fade included adding colors to the top (usually blond but also red, blue, or purple) or cutting designs into the back. These fanciful carvings included the continent of Africa, the Statue of Liberty, a girlfriend's name, or even Bart Simpson. Corporate logos, triangles, Batman symbols, wavy lines, initials, boxes, nicknames, slopes, valleys, and multicolored patches all appeared in fades. Little twists or dredlocs on the hair on top (often with the tips dyed blond or orange), cuts such as the Box (a very square fade), the Gumby (in which the hair on top is on a sideways-tilting slope), the shag, the Cameo, and the pompadour all had their moment. Each city, region, and even barbershop had its specialty or variation.

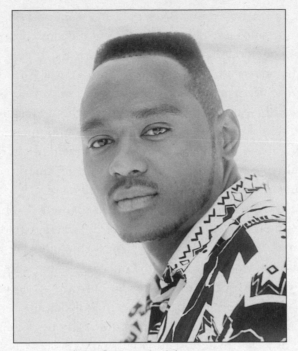

An eighties fade. © Hosea L. Johnson.

Needless to say, with so many styling options to choose from, young men were spending a lot of time at the barber. Some went as often as every five days, a marked change from the days of the Afro, when barber visits could be few and far between. Establishments like Joseph's Barber Shop in Washington, D.C., offered a budget plan for students because young men came in so often to keep their looks manicured.

The emergence of such a dizzying array of styles, most never before seen on the heads of Black youth in America, did not go unnoticed. Opinions on the cuts were often as colorful as the styles themselves. There was a contingent who believed these new looks were mere fanciful flights of youth intended strictly for the purpose of looking good and keeping up with the trends. Others believed the styles looked thuggish and pointed out the difficulty of securing gainful employment if you had a sloped, blond-tipped hairdo with Batman carved into the back. However, there were some, young and old, who pointed to these very same haircuts as an expression of Black pride, noting that it was the unique texture of Black hair that allowed it to be styled in these artful looks. Furthermore, the

Five Famous Men with Equally Famous Hair

AL SHARPTON—Some do it for fashion. Others for convenience. But the Reverend Al Sharpton did it for love—the love of soul singer James Brown. In 1981 Sharpton was to accompany Brown, who was his mentor and surrogate father, to the White House. But first Brown made a detour to visit the woman in Georgia who had styled his hair many times before. He wanted her to get Sharpton's locs to resemble his own, so they could look like father and son. Two decades later, Sharpton's press-and-curl look still persists.

Daring Afrocentrists and activists alike to tell him that a pro-Black leader can't rest his battle-weary head under curlers and a scarf at night, Sharpton has been fighting the good fight for as long as he's been wearing his now trademark coiffure. Permed and then curled into a bouffant (that has lost some of its height over the years), it is not a look often seen on the streets or in the courtrooms of New York City. And the likelihood for change is slim. Brown made his surrogate son promise he would wear his hair like that until the day Brown died. An emotional Sharpton agreed, and the rest is big hair history.

LITTLE RICHARD—Before Prince picked up a jar of relaxer and before Michael Jackson showed the world just how shiny one Black man could get his hair, there was Little Richard. He may have been denied credit for many of his firsts, but no one can deny that this singing, piano-playing musical genius from Macon, Georgia, is responsible for the curls, the gleam, and the outrageousness that a good conk can produce when coupled with setting lotion and a little imagination. Good golly, Miss Molly!

BOB MARLEY—Robert Nesta Marley, the Jamaican-born man who became an international star bringing reggae music to the world, will forever be the most famous dred. His natty dreds symbolized all that a world often filled with corruption and artifice could be—strong, independent, and self-defined. Author Alice Walker, who has worn her hair in dredlocs since the 1980s, once wrote, "Bob Marley is the person who taught me to trust the universe enough to respect my hair." As he shook his lion's mane, the confidence, the love, and the sheer commitment to Blackness and to Jah was in his every movement.

DON KING—Mr. King doesn't only have the monopoly on the world of professional box-ing; his most famous Don King Production sits right on top of his head and close to his heart. Ever since Troll dolls lost their trendy coolness and Lionel Richie went for the S-Curl, King's high-jinks hair is the longest-standing example of a man and his simple but unwavering love for an uncombed 'fro. According to Mr. King, his gravity-defying 'do is a showpiece from the heavenly spirits and not a random style. "It's an aura from God," King once told a reporter, one that suddenly appeared from up above. "I don't know why God has chosen me through my hair," his holiness declared. "It's a mystery." Perhaps the good Lord wasn't resting on the seventh day after all.

MR. T.—Before Mr. T., a mohawk hairstyle received very little respect outside the world of punk rock. But when this fool-pitying giant muscled his way into our national consciousness in 1982 as the preternaturally shiny foe of Sylvester "Rocky III" Stallone and then as B(ad) A(ss) Baracus on *The A-Team,* a shaved head, mountains of gold jewelry, and high-top sneakers fi-nally stood for something. What exactly? It's hard to say, but Mr. T. never strayed from his signature hairdo, which he insisted paid homage to his African Mandingo ancestors. And you thought it was just a gimmick.

HONORABLE MENTIONS

BUCKWHEAT—So much more than a character from *The Little Rascals,* this living 1930s stereotype—with mile-high hair that looks like it never made friends with a comb—has be-come the patron saint of bad hair days for Black America.

JESUS—If Jesus was the original Black man, as many believe, then his referenced flowing locs and lamb's-wool hair might have looked a lot like Bob Marley's glorious mane. Let the Church say Amen to the possibility.

variety of styles were created by Black people and were not an imitation of any cuts worn by other racial groups. Washington, D.C., image consultant Helen Moody was quoted in *The Washington Post* as saying that the styles "psychologically created a wonderful kind of brotherness. It's as if the haircuts have taken a place alongside the handshakes—there's almost like a kind of code that goes with them, an unspoken thing. . . . The brothers have got something that is their own, that can't be taken away from them the way that braids were taken from [Black women]." In fact, if any imitation was occurring, it was by White people who were trying to

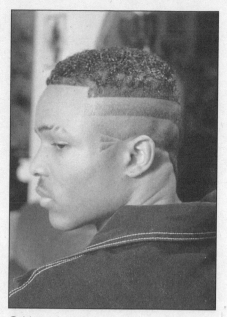

© Hosea L. Johnson.

copy these Black cuts. Rapper Vanilla Ice had a high-top fade with various designs cut into it that looked part Elvis, part Kid 'N Play. White hip-hop group 3rd Bass also wore fades. Many White youth who listened to hip-hop attempted to mimic the hairstyles they saw on their favorite rappers.

Free Fallin'

Black men were not the only ones doing never-before-tried things with their hair. African-American women also used the post-Afro days to experiment with daring hairstyles. With the new hair-care products such as mousse and gel, both White and Black women began experimenting with "big" hair, meaning hair with extreme volume. Oprah Winfrey's hair in the early days of her national talk show was a prime example of "big" African-American hair. Patti LaBelle's "wings" of hair, while not typical of anything except the singer's creative urges, also demonstrated the eighties propensity for playing with styling products to achieve never-before-seen styles.

The emergence of hip-hop also had an effect on the styling choices of young Black women. Younger African-American females could now turn

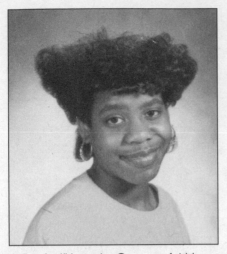

A "stacked" hairstyle. Courtesy of Akiba Solomon.

on music videos or look on their favorite album covers for hairstyles that reflected their generation and were worn by women who perhaps shared their socioeconomic background and lifestyle. "Black women rappers sport distinctively Black hairstyles . . . that ground them in a contemporary working-class Black youth aesthetic," wrote Tricia Rose. "They affirm Black female working-class cultural signs and experiences that are rarely depicted in American popular culture." Through these styles, hair was increasingly coming to be seen as a class divider. "In general, working-class and low-income Black girls and women were the hair trailblazers at this time," notes essayist and cultural critic Asali Solomon. "Middle- and upper-income blacks wore more conventional permed styles, where the emphasis was on the vertical length of the hair, as opposed to its ability to flout gravity and incorporate extravagant sculpting details. In this way, hair became somewhat a marker of class."

The cuts created by these "hair trailblazers" were asymmetric cuts, "wedges" or "stacks" (where the hair is cut into blunt angles, curled under and "stacked" upon one another), finger waves (where hair is slicked down to the head and an exaggerated ripple effect is added), and a spectacular use of color and hair dyes (such as temporary color that was sprayed on like hairspray to streak the hair red or blue). The list of styles was near endless, as each region of the country and specific cities put their own twist on a look and created a new variation. And, as with the men's looks, these styles often were created on the street level, and celebrities would adopt them. For example, when female rap group Salt 'N Pepa wore blond stacks they were not starting a trend, they were following it.

Regardless of how the styles started, the common thread with each of these looks was that they all required straight hair. Black women after the seventies largely turned away from natural hairstyles in their search for beauty and instead radicalized the perm to create straightened hair looks of dizzying variety and originality. These styles, with their height, often dazzling color, and in-your-face defiance of convention were the true "extreme" hairstyles of the era. Susan Bordo notes that at a time of color contact lenses and White women with deep tans and cornrows, beauty trends for Black and White women in the eighties were "seen as having . . . no political valance . . . and [no] cultural meaning . . . in the heterogeneous yet undifferentiated context of the things 'all' women do 'to be more attractive.'" Black women, younger Black women in particular, were once again wowing America with their hairstyles, but this time the needed accessory was a kit of Bone Strait Relaxer as opposed to an Afro pick.

The culmination of these arresting styles was the hair show. Hair shows, initially intended as industry conferences, originated in the sixties but peaked in popularity in the eighties. By this time they had evolved into hair-raising competitions, featuring the wildest creations that a hairstylist could envision. Events such as the biannual four-day event Hair Wars in Detroit brought stylists from around the country to create visions of grandeur via the hair. An *InStyle* article on the shows quotes a beautician explaining, "Hair is like food: You've got the same basic groups, but you can do so many different things with it."

Unbeweavable!

One day Oprah Winfrey got up on her stage and started outing people. Famous people. Janet Jackson. Guilty. Diana Ross. Really guilty. Winfrey wasn't divulging sexual secrets; she was talking about hair. On national television the country's most popular talk-show host—who once admitted she'd always wanted hair that swung from side to side—was announcing who in Hollywood wore a weave. Short of revealing who sported breast implants, this was one of the riskiest things for Oprah to do. There were few Black models who did not wear weaves, but many people in mainstream America had been fooled. Naomi Campbell? Weave. Iman? Weave. Tyra Banks? Weave. Watching television through the late eighties and early nineties was like viewing a who's who of weave wearers. A staggering majority of the women in music videos were weaved. Lisa Bonet's hair changed length for almost every episode of her *Cosby* spin-off, *A Different World*. Janet Jackson went from cute Cleo with a short permed bun on *Fame* to a "Miss Jackson if you're nasty" superstar with a long, curly mane.

These celebrities were not the only ones wearing weaves. "Sisters love the weave!" *Essence* magazine declared in 1990. Although women had been wearing them since the sixties (and wigs and hair attachments predate the Civil War), the weaves of the late eighties and nineties were major improvements over their predecessors. Less bulky than earlier versions, these modern weaves were also available in a wider range of colors and textures (straight, wet and wavy, superwavy, kinky), thus maximizing the chances that no one would know that someone's hair was actually fake. The add-on tresses, often human hair but sometimes yak hair or synthetic, was attached by one of numerous methods. In the most popular technique, the weave wearer's own hair would be cornrowed, and then "tracks" (strips of hair sewn onto netting) were sewn directly onto the braided hair. There was also "bonding" (when tracks were glued to the hair at the roots) and "singeing" (using heat, synthetic hair was machine pressed onto the natural hair). The process, which was obviously best left to a professional, could cost anywhere from two hundred to fifteen hundred dollars.

Models claimed to get weaves to protect their own hair, which was liable to be damaged by all the abuse it took on shoots from hairdressers often unaccustomed to styling African-American hair. Tyra Banks remembers once doing five fashion shows every day for a month early in her career and the havoc it wreaked on her hair. At one show the stylist wanted her to have an Afro, so they crimped, teased, and sprayed Banks's hair. At the next stop she had mounds of beeswax put in her hair to simulate dredlocs. Next, the dredloc style was combed out and her hair hot-curled to achieve a curly look. "There was no shampooing or conditioning between all of this," Banks recalls. "It's no wonder my hair was falling out in clumps." Soon after, the supermodel began wearing weaves and hair attachments to protect her locs.

Many other women, models as well as regular folks, saw weaves as the way to have versatile looks and just-step-out-of-bed-and-go hair. Through the use of weaves, the long-standing Black problem of not having long hair was effectively solved for many. But while weaves were everywhere, they were generally looked down upon. The same men who would compliment a woman on her long hair would look scornfully on the idea that it could be a weave. Baby boomer Samuel Roosevelt speaks for a lot of men when he says that a woman can do anything she wants with her hair as long as it's not a wig or a weave. "Because it's not yours," he states emphatically. "You're trying to be something that you're not, and that's very, very unattractive." Police captain Craig Price adds, "It's the same thing as wearing falsies [bra inserts]."

At the same time that weaves were gaining popularity, so was another look that required hair add-ons. Braid extensions required added hair that was braided into a person's own hair, thereby creating a braid that could stay in for a long period of time. Braid styles were waist long or pixie short, and the thickness of braids went from micro-thin to a thick width popularly known as "dookie" braids. Some braiders worked out of hair salons (where styles could cost over three hundred dollars), yet most women opted to go to the home of a woman who braided hair to get their styles. An underground, unlicensed "kitchen salon" system blossomed that continues today. Female African immigrants who lived in cities like New York and Boston were in high demand to re-create some of the styles that were worn in the Motherland. Women of all classes, ages, and locales wore the varying braid looks, heralding them as a way to have get-up-and-go hair that could face the rain, the gym, and the beach, yet was based in an aesthetic that dated back to pre–slave trade Africa. And as with its cousin, the weave, these braids gave many women long, movable hair for the first time in their lives.

Why did this obsession with long hair suddenly resurface with such force? One could say that the desire never went away but simply lay dormant during the Black Pride movement. Another major factor in the new obsession for long and straight was the introduction of the Black music video via *Video Music Box*, the main viewing outlet. *Video Music Box* debuted nationally in the late eighties, and for the first time America was barraged all day and all night with images of Black women on their televisions. The majority of these Black women, who overwhelmingly appeared in the videos as dancers wearing outfits that looked more like stripper gear, were light-skinned and had very long, very "movable" hair.

The late sixties and seventies "Black is beautiful" movement was intended to liberate Blacks from enslavement to the concepts of "good" and "bad" hair. Yet as the eighties progressed, it appeared that instead of being the beginning of change, those decades had been the exception to the aesthetic status quo. Beauty ideals remained firmly entrenched in a Eurocentric image of long, "swinging" hair. The only real difference was that the mainstream White press was finally including Black women in the national dialogue about what constituted beauty. It was in the eighties that Revlon introduced its "Most Beautiful Women in the World" ad campaign, the first mass-market campaign in which supermodels of all races were featured alongside one another. No longer relegated to the "ethnic" ads, the Somalian supermodel Iman could be featured next to Cindy Crawford; Dutch-African Louise Veyant or African-American Karen Alexander could be seen alongside the White French model Estelle. Vanessa Williams was crowned Miss America in 1984, and although some Blacks pointed out that she was light-skinned and had long hair and blue-green eyes, it was still remarkable that an African-American winner and runner-up (Suzette Charles) were selected in the pageant that had once been a bastion of "wholesome" (i.e., White) American-ness. Still, as sociologist Ann DuCille notes in her book *Skin Trade*, "Unless I have missed a few pageants along the way . . . the hairstyles of the Black women crowned Miss America or of the colored women crowned Miss Universe have differed little from those of the White contestants. . . . We have yet to see Miss America or Black Miss Universe with an Afro or cornrows or dredlocs."

As African-American casting agents sought out light-skinned, long-haired women for music videos, and White casting agents looked for Black models with "refined" (European) features, voices of discontent could be heard on the sidelines. *Essence* magazine remained committed to featuring models of all skin tones. Poets and writers such as Audre Lorde, Lisa Jones, and Gwendolyn Brooks continued to question the pervasiveness of a Eurocentric beauty ideal in their work. Afrocentrists celebrated an African-based aesthetic and promoted natural hairstyles and headwraps. In 1988 African-American filmmaker Spike Lee released *School Daze*, and Black and White audiences watched his take on hair issues and color complexes as it was played out on a fictitious Black college campus. The film pitted the light-skinned, long-haired students (the 'wannabees') against the darker, nappy-headed ones (the 'jigaboos'). In a pivotal scene, the women from each group have a standoff in Madam Re-Re's beauty parlor, singing "Straight and Nappy," with the chorus "Go on I swear, see if I care, good and bad hair." The song, as well as the film, brought to light demons that many Blacks hoped had been exorcised.

Dred-ed Appeal

Before the influence of hip-hop and the emergence of music videos had an impact on Black hair, reggae music began gaining popularity in America,

and with it came the introduction of dredlocs. Dredlocs, the style popularized by Rastafarians, are the result of hair that has not been combed and
has grown into ropelike pieces. The word *dredlocs* signifies, according to
Tracy Nicholas's *Rastafari: A Way of Life,* "unholy peoples' fear of the
dreadful power of the holy." The name derives from the days of the slave
trade. When Africans emerged from the slave ships after months spent in
conditions adverse to any personal hygiene, Whites would declare the matted hair that had grown out of their kinky unattended locs to be "dreadful." (For that reason, many today wearing the style choose to drop the *a* in
dredloc to remove all negative connotations.) The Rastafarian religion adopted the hairstyle out of admiration and reverence for the fearless resistance of the Kikuyu soldiers of the Mau Mau rebellion in Kenya, who wore
their hair in the style while fighting British colonizers in the 1950s. The
Rasta commitment to dredlocs is also based on an interpretation of three
scriptures from the Bible (Leviticus 19:27, Leviticus 21:5, and Numbers
6:5), in which it is stated that hair should not be cut on the head or the face.
Rastafarians see dreds as "an indisputable racial characteristic," meaning
that only Black people, because of the texture of their hair, can grow them
without resorting to unusual means. Simply by washing the hair and letting it be, Black people can end up with dredlocs.

As reggae music, and especially the music of Jamaican Rastafarian Bob
Marley, became popular outside the Caribbean, dredlocs were introduced
to the rest of the world. Many of those in the United States who grew the
style in the early to mid-eighties did so because they were dabbling in
Rastafarianism. Yet it is the story of a Philadelphia organization called
MOVE that exemplifies how many Americans, both Black and White, initially saw dreds. Among significant segments of the population, the style
was not appreciated but was seen instead as unhygienic, militant, and aggressive.

MOVE, originally called the American Christian Movement for Life,
was founded in the early seventies by a man named John Africa (his birth
name was Vincent Leaphard). In keeping with their leader's philosophy of
getting back to nature, MOVE members, who all took the last name Africa, were encouraged to eat only raw vegetables and were prohibited from
using soap, electric heat, and other inventions of a modern society. MOVE
followers were also required to wear their hair in dredlocs as a symbol of
their overall commitment to living a natural life.

The members of MOVE came to national attention on May 13, 1985, when the Philadelphia police dropped a bomb on the rooftop bunker of their compound and then let it burn. The resulting fire destroyed sixty-one homes in the neighborhood and left eleven people (including five children) dead and two hundred fifty-three people, most unconnected to MOVE, homeless. Of the thirteen MOVE members in the compound at the time, only Ramona Johnson Africa, thirty, and thirteen-year-old Birdie Africa survived. Although it was not until the 1985 tragedy that the rest of America learned of the radical group, they had been well known since the seventies to Philadelphians. MOVE members and sympathizers of the group were easy to pick out of the average Philadelphia crowd because of their dredlocs. At a time when reggae music and Rastafarianism were just becoming known outside the Caribbean, Philadelphians typically associated dredlocs with this fringe group. And the associations were not positive. MOVE members were seen as aggressive, violent, unclean, and uncivilized by the media and many citizens, and their hair was used to support these characterizations. Like the bald styles worn by white supremacist skinheads, dredlocs became inextricably connected to the "problem" that was MOVE. "Dreds were associated with everything about MOVE members every time they were mentioned, and none of it was positive," recalls lifetime Philadelphia resident Stephanie Williams. "You never heard anything good about them. It wasn't until Bob Marley and Rastafarians that there was an alternative view about dredlocs. They weren't negative. It was more of a curiosity, like 'How did they get their hair like that?'"

Interestingly, Birdie and the other children of MOVE were aware of how their hair set them apart from others. In an interview Birdie gave on the tenth anniversary of the fire that killed his playmates and their parents, he told about a time when he and the other MOVE children wanted to run away but feared that their locs would give them away: "So Tree cut our hair. She must have been about ten or eleven then. We were serious. But [once] we got our hair cut, we didn't know where to go. . . . When the adults came for us and saw we had cut our hair, they didn't say anything to us for a couple of days."

Aside from MOVE members, dreds were starting to be worn by some other Blacks in America, particularly artists and intellectuals. Much like the Black bohemians in New York's Greenwich Village who wore their hair unstraightened in the late fifties and early sixties, these were people who were using their hair as a further expression of their liberal politics and their decision not to buy into the ideals and aesthetics of mainstream American society. Graffiti-artist-cum-neoexpressionist Jean-Michel Basquiat, activist and educator Angela Davis, author Alice Walker, and singer Tracy Chapman were four high-profile examples of early dred wearers in the United States. Often these people saw dredlocs less as a style than as a manifestation of certain ideals and beliefs. Alice Walker, in a 1989 *Essence* profile, said, "Once you dred your hair, everything falls into place. I could not have written *The Temple of My Familiar* with straight hair, what I call 'oppressed hair.' . . . I would like to say to other Black women looking at me and my hair . . . You don't have to be afraid. . . . You can just be free."

Dreds soon spread to other segments of the population. Some rappers, many of them with roots in the Caribbean, started wearing the style. Soon it became incorporated into the range of hairstyles of young hip-hop America, but usually with innovative twists, such as dreds only on top or with the ends dyed blond. Early nineties talk-show host Bertrice Berry ignored the directives of her show's executives to cut her hair and became the first African-American television personality with the style. Whoopi Goldberg's dredlocs made her Hollywood's "antibeauty," as she eschewed all conventional notions of what an attractive movie star could look like. *Cosby* star Lisa Bonet melded two popular trends of the time and wore a dred style that was actually hair attachments.

The Americanization of dredlocs, in which the style was removed from its biblical, religious, Rastafarian roots, was seen as something akin to blasphemy by many. In a 1991 *Essence* editorial, "The Dreaded Decision," writer and dred-wearer Naadu Blankson recalled "one Jamaican girlfriend who told me in no uncertain terms that 'Yankees dat dread dem har bodda me.'" African-American community philanthropist Kofi Taha explains, "The main problem is the absence of any of the original spiritual process that the decision to dred once implied, or any of the political action that gave the style that name. What is learned when you go to the salon to get your dreds done? What struggle is being waged when locs become fashionable? What happened to the 'dreaded man' that scared those British soldiers out of their mind?" Taha's sentiments echo those of the multitudes who felt that the fashionizing of the style was similar to the commodification that went on when Bo Derek wore braids. When *Essence* magazine ran how-to articles on the style, offhandedly noting how it was "popularized in the Carib-

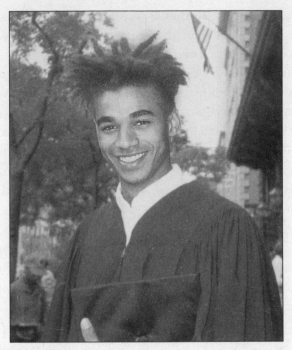

Locs get trendy in America, 1991. From the authors' collection.

bean to a reggae beat and a Rastafarian philosophy," a number of readers wrote in to lambast the publication for having "crucified the dread!"

The assertion that African-Americans with dreds were wearing the style only as a fashion oversimplifies the situation. First, even as a fashion statement the embracing of dredlocs was significant in that it was a negation of all things Black hair was "supposed" to look like, namely straight and neat. Second, many were wearing the look as a way to connect visibly to their African roots by celebrating the Blackness of their hair, hair that was able to grow into such a style. Last, Rastafarian assertions that Black Americans were co-opting "their" style are based on questionable logic. Rastafarians did not "invent" dredlocs; they adopted the look from Kenyan soldiers, but the style dates to before the fifth century, when Bahatowie priests of the Ethiopian Coptic Church locked their hair. The sadhus, a nomadic group of Hindu holy men, have worn their hair in this way since the pre-Christian centuries as a symbol of a covenant between themselves and Shiva, the god of destruction and regeneration. From Japan's Rasta-Buddhists to

Maori warriors in New Zealand, various groups have adopted dredlocs as a style endowed with symbolism, reverence, and aesthetic meaning. It is a hairstyle over which no group can claim ownership.

Yet and still, dredlocs and their commodification in Black American culture made an interesting statement about the evolution of Black hair. Was it possible for Blacks to appropriate something that was Black in its essence? While debates and opinions raged on, the style was spreading to other groups outside the African-American community. By the early nineties, particularly in California, Whites and Asians had begun to wear the style. A Venice Beach hair salon, Papers Scissors Rock, managed by Japanese-American Masao Miyashiro, charged two hundred dollars to begin dreds for people in 1994. Only 15 percent of their clientele was African-American. Some were Asian, particularly Japanese tourists, but most were white bicycle messengers, surfers, and other young white Californians. Papers Scissors Rock was relatively inexpensive compared with some other salons that specialized in dreding hair and charged up to a thousand dollars. The cost was so high because of the time and effort that went into getting non-nappy hair to loc. It presents a more daunting problem than napping up unkinky hair to make an Afro. Some solutions for locing unwilling hair include washing it with beeswax or baking soda, coating the hair with a chemical relaxer to break down the structure of the hair, using Krazy Glue to form the knots around which the dreds are coiled, and putting toothpicks into the newly formed locs to encourage them to grow downward. Some people simply had extensions of dreded hair added to their own.

As with Bo Derek's wearing of cornrows, some Black people were not pleased with non-Blacks wearing dredlocs. "I try not to care and to think to each his own," says twenty-something Brooklyn writer and former dred wearer Karen Good. "But somewhere deep inside of me, it just doesn't sit well." Reasons cited for disliking the look on Whites and Asians run the gamut from simply being aesthetically displeasing to making a mockery of a time-honored, culturally significant tradition. However, the adoption of the style can also be seen as a way of challenging the norms of acceptability. Kofi Taha explains, "Usually White folks with dreds are rebelling against more than just aesthetic norms, and that's a good first step toward a larger consciousness for some people."

Afro Chic

In March 1994 the urban entertainment magazine *Vibe* featured a fashion story titled "Free Angela: Actress Cynda Williams as Angela Davis, a Fashion Revolutionary." The layout was termed a *docufashion* because it featured modern clothes mimicking the look of the seventies. In the story Williams wears an enormous Afro wig and in some pictures a see-through minidress. There are courtroom scenes and pictures of her getting arrested. *Vibe* even reprints the FBI poster but with Williams as Davis. While the editors of *Vibe* most likely saw their story as a way to pay homage to a time in Black history, Angela Davis felt differently. She saw the recreation of the FBI poster, the poster used to hunt her down for a murder charge, as "the most blatant example of the way the particular history of my legal case is emptied of all content so that it can serve as a commodified backdrop for advertising." In her book *The Angela Y. Davis Reader* she writes, "It never occurred to me that the same 'revolutionary' image I then sought to camouflage with glamour [when she was underground] would be turned, a generation later, into glamour and nostalgia."

Davis's concerns over the manner in which her case, and her hairstyle, had been wiped clean of their meaning and politics were not shared by the masses. By the middle of the 1990s, more than two decades after Black Pride and Afros had appeared, Black people were overwhelmingly taking the liberty of wearing their hair however they wanted and basically hoping that their employers didn't complain. Little appeared to be sacred anymore. With the continued growth of a Black popular culture that now included film, television shows, music videos, and magazines, African-Americans were not only finally exercising a higher degree of control over the images that they presented but were able to decide how to manipulate the meaning behind an image. Many saw it as a time of freedom of choice for Blacks. Yet as the twentieth century closed in on its final years, African-Americans still had many hair skeletons lurking in their collective closet.

6

The Burden of Proof:
Explaining Black Hair Culture

Amy Thomas* was used to being the token. Growing up in the suburbs of a midsize Midwestern city, attending private schools from kindergarten through college, and working in a corporate environment in Manhattan had prepared Thomas for a permanent position as the Black cultural ambassador to White America. Over the years she had developed stock answers on the subjects White people most needed answers to—everything from ashy skin to chitterlings—and always managed to avoid insult or conflict. Still, nothing in Amy Thomas's mostly White upbringing spared her the shock and subsequent epiphany that occurred one day in 1995.

Amy was working diligently in her office at one of the largest advertising agencies in New York. She had just finished hanging up a new calendar

*Note: In this chapter most names have been changed.

that had been sent to her by a former client. Suddenly Amy was interrupted by one of her coworkers, a tall honey-blond White woman, originally from the South. Charlotte and Amy were by no means friends, but they were friendly and often gossiped together at lunchtime. When Charlotte entered Amy's office she burst out laughing, hand over her mouth in mock horror as she read the wording on Amy's new calendar. "Creme of Nature!" she cried aloud. "What is that?" Amy was confused. "What do you mean what is it? It's shampoo. It's made by Revlon." As tears of laughter began streaming down Charlotte's cheeks, Amy quickly retraced her childhood. Creme of Nature was always there. It was the shampoo her whole family had always used religiously. What was causing this woman to find it so funny? She soon got her answer. "Creme of Nature," Charlotte sputtered. "It sounds like an exotic way to say [her voice lowered to a whisper] semen." Now it was Amy's turn to be disgusted. Before long every White person in her department had stepped into her office for a laugh over the kinky shampoo calendar.

When Amy went home that evening, the day's events replayed in her mind. Did the words *creme of nature* really evoke such lurid images? Maybe, but it was hard to associate the name with anything more than hair products. She felt that her coworkers had simply gone too far. Who cared if they had never heard of the product before? That's when it hit her. None of those people in her office had any knowledge of the shampoos made specifically for Black people or probably of any other "ethnic" hair product for that matter. It was like a revelation for Amy. She realized that when it came to hair, White people were completely unaware of what really went on in Black America. Before she fell asleep that night, Amy made a mental note to add Black hair culture to her growing list of phenomena to explain to the rest of the world.

Black Hair Culture 101

America was built on the myth of the melting pot, but despite the efforts of the powers that be, the ingredients never fully blended. At best there is a patchwork quilt of various ethnic groups struggling to live peacefully with one another while something called "mainstream culture"—it looks like a Norman Rockwell painting, sounds like a George Gershwin musical, and tastes like Chef Boyardee—is offered up as the national example. The pervasiveness of what bell hooks terms this "dull dish that is mainstream White culture" has succeeded in keeping many people unaware of the diversity surrounding them, including the unique culture of Black hair.

Culture is a sticky subject and can be interpreted in many ways. Anthropologists define culture as the strategies by which humans adapt to their natural environment. The many aspects of human adaptation—including language, technology, traditions, values, and social organization—are all identifiable components of the culture of Black hair in America. And although academics and laypeople alike might doubt the assertion that a culture specific to Black hair exists, the truth is self-evident.

In the United States, where the aesthetic norms are overwhelmingly based on a White European standard, Black people with any variation of kinky tresses are immediately cast as "others" in mainstream beauty culture. Since the first Black slaves set foot on the beaches of Jamestown, Virginia, their hair-raising strategies to adapt and fit in have been passed on from generation to generation. This was the beginning of Black hair culture in America. And what of those Black Americans born without the follicular stamp of Negro heritage? By virtue of their African ancestry in this one-drop-rule nation, even these kink-free, straight-haired Black citizens have a confirmed place in the social order of Black hair culture.

Hot Combs and Hair Grease: The Language and Technology of Hair

From day one, Black children are indoctrinated into the intricate culture of hair. Vocabulary words like *grease, kitchen* (the hair at the nape of the neck, not the room in the house), and *touch-up* are ones a Black child hears at a very early age and needs to learn in order to fully participate in the Black hair lifestyle. Phrases like *nappy-headed, tender-headed,* and *turn back* aren't so much taught as they are absorbed into the growing lexicon of a young Black mind. Before a Black child is even born, relatives speculate over the texture of hair that will cover the baby's head, and the loaded adjectives "good" and "bad" are already in the air.

Keeping in mind that culture is passed on from one generation to the next, the prevalence of the "good" hair/"bad" hair dichotomy present in modern Black hair culture is not surprising. Black men and women from all parts of the country recall hearing the labels everywhere from the playground at school to the sermons at church. Definitions range from the serious to the sardonic. "Good hair is like that silky black shit that them Indian girls be havin'. It's wavy, it's got a little curl goin' on, and looks real fly 'cause she can grow it out real long. . . . Good hair is anything that's not crazy-ass woolly, lookin' like some pickaninny out the bush," declares Joicelyn Chambers, a New York City dancer.

"I remember growing up with a girl named Wanda who had long, wavy hair," says Long Island native Patricia Watson. "People always referred to her as 'Wanda with the good hair.'" Saundra Adams, who grew up in the San Francisco Bay Area, comments, "I have a best friend who is still insistent that I have 'good' hair and she has 'bad' hair. As a matter of fact, the only argument that we've had in our eleven-year friendship was over the insistence of this concept." Euphemisms for good hair also have to be learned, like "Indian hair," "curly hair," or "nice hair." Likewise, there are other monikers for "bad" hair like "peasy" (as in, the hair is so tightly curled it looks like peas) and "nappy." Cynthia Racks remembers, "I was about seven when I overheard someone say that I had 'coarse' hair and I thought that meant 'Wow! I like her hair.' I found out not long afterwards that coarse wasn't a compliment." Kathryn Benson, a young woman who grew up in the eighties in Florida, says she was taught that bad hair was "that really kinky, curly, 'woolish' type of natural hair." Thankfully, there have been efforts to strike these archaic classifications from Black hair vernacular or at the very least redefine them. "I was going to a local hairdresser," says Maya Cole of an experience in North Carolina. "She corrected me when I talked about my hair as being 'bad' hair. She told me that if you have hair covering your head, and it holds a style well, that is 'good' hair."

Learning the language of Black hair culture goes hand in hand with understanding the technology. As the tools created to manipulate Black hair advance, the language continues to expand. The original tool of Black hair culture has to be the ancient hand-carved African comb, better known in America as the Afro pick. This wide-toothed invention has served as the prototype for modern utensils—from blow-dryer attachments to regular combs—used by Black people all over the world. Other equipment can be grouped according to function in the following categories: straighteners, styling tools, moisturizers, pomades (also known as grease), and accessories.

Familiarity with the tools and fluidity in the language of Black hair culture does not automatically qualify a person as a member of the club, however. Certain rituals and rites of passage must also be experienced.

Rituals and Rites of Passage

CHILDHOOD

The care of Black hair requires patience, time, and a healthy dose of creativity. In its natural state, kinky hair tends to be extremely dry, very fragile, and generally requires less washing than finer textured hair. Little Black girls usually get their hair washed anywhere from once a week to once a month, and then it must be arranged into some sort of style or it will be nearly impossible to manage until the next washing. Regardless of the desired look—from Afro puffs to intricate cornrows to Shirley Temple Curls—the hair has to be combed out, a small section at a time, and blow-drying is often necessary. For many Blacks, memories of early hair-care rituals are unforgettable, for reasons both bad and good. Feminist author and social critic bell hooks describes pleasurable hair-straightening days from her childhood in her memoir *Bone Black*. "We are six girls who live in a house together. . . . We sit in the kitchen and wait our turn for the hot comb, wait to sit in the chair by the stove, smelling grease, feeling the heat warm our scalp like a sticky hot summer sun." Regardless of age, both old and young reach back to hair rituals as seductive memories. "As a child my mother washed my hair every Saturday afternoon for church on Sunday," remembers Monisha Franklin, who grew up in Ann Arbor, Michigan. "Since it took so long, she used to give me dates to eat while she talked to me and washed my hair in the kitchen sink. I used to sit on the counter and lean back over the sink while she washed and told me stories and I ate those dates. To this day, I eat dates and feel cared for."

Men too get to take part in these memorable hair bonding experiences. Roger Stanton, a New York–based journalist, says his most positive hair memories are of his paternal grandmother braiding his and his brother's hair. "She only did it twice," says Stanton, who was a teenager at the time. "We let it stay in overnight, then unbraided it. It gave my brother and I these massive Afros, which at the time [the late seventies] was incredibly cool."

Black Hair Glossary

Nappy—Word used to describe tight kinky Black hair. Each individual kinky curl is considered a nap, thus a head full of Black hair is considered nappy.

Hot Comb—A comb originally made of iron that is heated over a flame, then combed through kinky hair to make it straight. Also referred to as a straightening comb or pressing comb.

"Go Back"/"Turn Back"—Phrase usually used in despair when hair straightened by a hot comb or other heat-based methods reverts back to its naturally kinky state. Black hair usually turns back when it comes in contact with moisture of any kind.

The Kitchen—the patch of hair at the nape of the neck. This hair is usually the nappiest and most difficult to get straight with the hot comb (see above).

Hair Grease—A generic term for almost any moisturizing product used either to make the hair shine (i.e., a pomade), to make a hot comb slide through without burning the hair, or to lubricate the scalp. Often comes in rainbow colors like blue, green, and pink.

Relaxer—A chemical treatment that turns kinky or tightly curled hair straight. Effects generally last for six to eight weeks, then a new relaxer must be applied to the newly grown-in hair. Also colloquially referred to as a perm.

New Growth—Phrase used by relaxer wearers to reference the hair that grows in after the relaxer is applied (e.g. "I got a perm last month, but I already have two inches of new growth so I need to get a touch-up").

Touch-Up—Usually a relaxer that is only applied to new growth (see above) (e.g., "Ooohh, my roots are getting nappy. I need a touch-up").

Texturizer—A relaxer that is left in the hair for only a short amount of time, just long enough to loosen the curl pattern slightly. (See Chris Rock, post-1997, or Sean "Puffy" Combs.)

Cornrows—A hairstyle of African origin achieved by sectioning hair and braiding it tightly against the scalp.

Dredlocs—What happens when nappy hair is left to its own devices. Sometimes achieved by twisting the hair first, then leaving it alone until the individual strands of hair begin to loc around each other to form a ropelike appearance. Does not require wax or glue or other foreign objects. Does not requre abstaining from regular hair hygiene, i.e., washing and conditioning.

Hard-headed—Term usually used to describe children who can withstand the pulling, tugging, and detangling process of getting their hair combed without crying.

Tender-headed—Opposite of hard-headed (see above).

Picky-headed—Derogatory adjective usually employed by an older generation to imply that one's hair does not look neat and may be sticking up all over one's head.

For many Black children, the time spent under the knowing hands of a mother, grandmother, or older sibling as they grease the scalp, then comb, braid, or twist the hair yields some of the most cherished moments of each day. "I remember when my cousin—who is extremely talented and creative—would braid my hair when I was a kid and she would come up with so many unique styles and patterns," says Shanna Little, reminiscing about her most positive hair experiences. "I would always get compliments. I felt like a peacock." Says Marcia Gillespie, editor-in-chief of *Ms.* magazine, "I think part of the stories that bind us together as Black [people] are our hair stories. I just look forward to the time when the hair stories won't be as traumatic."

Unfortunately, for many Black people childhood hair memories are tinged with bitterness and pain, a bad omen for a positive future relationship with one's own tresses. "I remember my mother picking out my hair

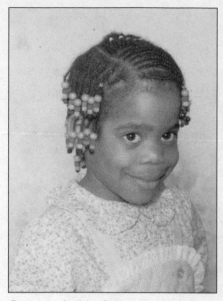

Courtesy of Akiba Solomon.

with an Afro pick every day," recalls Anthony Riggins. "My god, it hurt. I hated it because she was so forceful." A similar comment comes from Lynn Bracey: "When I was a child I hated to get my hair done. My mother would pull and swat me if I moved too much. She always seemed to burn me with that straightening comb."

The first date with "that straightening comb"—for some it stands as a rite of passage, for others it was the beginning of a painful relationship. "For each of us getting our hair pressed is an important ritual," bell hooks writes. "It is not a sign of our longing to be White. It is not a sign of our quest to be beautiful. We are girls. It is a sign of our desire to be women." In order to straighten the hair with a hot comb, the hair has to be clean, dry, and tangle-free. Some sort of pressing oil or grease is applied to condition the hair as well as to make it smooth and shiny. On contact with the comb, the grease will often make a sizzling sound, not unlike bacon frying in a cast-iron skillet. No matter how steady the person doing the hot-combing is, there is always the danger of hitting a trouble spot like an ear, a forehead, or the back of the neck with the red-hot piece of metal. Jamie White grew up in the eighties, and some of her worst memories revolve around the hot comb. "I would have to sit for thirty minutes to an hour being scared," she says. "It's not that my mom burned me often, but those few times she burned my ear really made an impression on me. I would flinch whenever I heard the sizzle of the grease."

When hair-care manufacturers introduced kinder, gentler relaxers especially formulated for young people in the early 1980s, many parents and children were overjoyed at the prospect of retiring the hot comb. The kiddie relaxer was touted as a pain-free alternative to the hot comb. "Relaxing should always be this gentle . . . As gentle as your love," read the ad copy for Dark & Lovely's Beautiful Beginnings children's relaxer. Once a girl has her hair permed, it stays relatively straight, even on contact with mois-

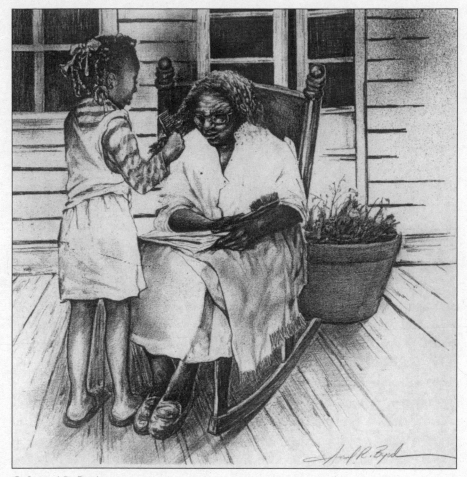

© Samuel R. Byrd.

ture. Make no mistake, permed hair still requires a lot of time and maintenance efforts (washing, blow-drying, conditioning), but infinitely less than unpermed hair. "Both my daughters (age eleven and eighteen) have relaxers and it's partly because of our lifestyle," explains Mary Lewis, a bank manager. "It's really more about the convenience of being able to wash it as much as you want."

Some parents are not eager to see their young daughters become a "slave to the chemicals," for reasons varying from hair health to lingering sixties "Black is beautiful" nostalgia. "I had to beg my mother to let me get my first perm when I was twelve," says writer Lauren Epps, twenty-six.

"All my friends had gotten perms, my cousin had a perm, and I wanted one too. But my mother, who used to wear a big Afro in the sixties and seventies, had no intention of letting me permanently straighten my hair."

The hesitation on the part of concerned parents is definitely warranted when it comes to the potential danger to the hair. If a child gets a perm at an early age, the caustic nature of the chemicals can damage the hair and/or scalp and permanently alter the texture, length, and volume of any future growth. In addition, the perm must be touched up every six to eight weeks, or severe breakage occurs where the new hair meets the relaxed hair. Whether the touch-up is done at a salon or at home, the maintenance can get rather costly. Children aren't always in favor of perms either. "Sometimes it would burn or itch," remembers eleven-year-old Monica Lewis, who believes the reason she got her first perm when she was eight years old was that her hair was too much work for her mother to handle.

Some people may wonder why parents would inflict the torture of the hot comb or a chemical relaxer on their young children, and the usual reply would fall somewhere between convenience and acceptability. It is never an easy answer, but adapting to America's visual norms often makes it easier for Black hair to move through White culture without causing a disturbance. The first time Black hair intersects with White people is a telling experience most people will never forget. "When I was in first grade I went to an after-school program with my hair in Afro puffs," says Kim Watson, who grew up in the seventies as one of only a handful of Blacks in a small town in Ohio. "The kids from another school called me 'Mickey Mouse,' and this quickly degenerated into 'nigger.' I wanted desperately to get rid of signs of my blackness, so I asked to get my hair relaxed." While not every experience is as traumatic as Watson's, the feeling of "otherness" as it relates to hair is one most Black people in America can identify with and recognize.

Black children, especially those who live in integrated neighborhoods and have friends of other ethnicities, realize early in life that their hair makes them different. Images they see on television and in their friends' homes prove that Black hair isn't like White hair. White people do not typically use hot combs to make their hair straight; they don't put oils and grease in their hair to make it shine; they usually wash it more often than once a week; and it does not take as long to get it into a satisfactory style. Something as innocuous as a slumber party—when all the other girls can just jump in the shower and the Black girl has to ask for a shower cap—can be an uncomfortable and awkward experience. It can make summer camp a downright nightmare. "When I went to Camp Minakani in northern Wisconsin, all the other girls in my cabin wanted to know why I didn't wash my hair every day," recalls Amy Thomas. "They acted like the fact that I put grease in my hair at night before I braided it was a disgusting, freaky thing. I felt so embarrassed I just stopped taking care of my hair for the rest of the summer. I actually felt better having my hair look dry and messy than having those girls think I was doing something gross."

School is often the first place Black children learn survival skills when it comes to their hair. They are forced to defend it, explain it, and often make excuses for it as White students and teachers remain unaware of their inner turmoil. "Being the only Black child in class in my elementary school, White kids were always awed at the texture of my hair," remembers Anthony Riggins. "There were definite insecurities I had because these wretched kids would want to touch it to see what it felt like. I don't know how many times I would just glare at them, with eyes that said, 'I'm not a dog.'" Even an innocuous event like having school pictures taken can make Black children hyperaware of the difference between their hair and everybody else's. When the teachers distribute those little fine-toothed black plastic combs so students can tidy up their hair, they never realize those flimsy instruments would never make it through a head of kinks and curls. So as not to draw attention to themselves, some children go so far as to take the comb and go through the motions of combing, hoping none of the other students notice the deception.

Another elementary school incident sure to test the mettle of young Black minds is when the inevitable lice epidemic breaks out. A typical reaction involves equal parts trepidation and pride. When all the students have to line up and get their hair picked over by the school nurse, many Black children feel confident that they'll be in the clear, based on the widely believed myth that Black people cannot get lice. Countless Black mothers assure their children that the little white creatures can't navigate their kinky, curly tresses or that hair grease makes Black hair inhospitable to lice. On the other hand, the trauma of having a White nurse or school volunteer poking around in their hair with a Q-Tip can be downright unnerving to a Black child because the nurse is often unaccustomed to the feel of their hair. Heaven forbid she comment aloud about the distinctive texture or the generous amount of hair grease being used for a high-gloss shine. Then the nurse continues to mess up the student's hairstyle, which cannot simply be patted back in place, so the child has to go through the rest of the day looking unkempt. Though embarrassing and sometimes painful, these trials are the ways young Black children mature in the life cycle of Black hair culture. Not much unlike the physical initiation rituals young men must go through in the New Guinea Highlands, surviving in mainstream culture with Black hair is like that insightful old refrain: What doesn't kill you makes you stronger.

The attitudes within the Black community regarding hair, some would argue, are far more damaging to a child's self-esteem and beauty image than the ignorance of mainstream White culture. For every story of a Black child like Kim Watson, who was taunted by White children about her Afro puffs, there is another story of a Black child tormented by her own family members or other Black friends. "I was a young girl with coarse hair," says Ashley Canady. "My brother and his friends would often tease me about it. Once the neighbor's cousin came to visit and she called me 'nippie nippie nap neck,' and that name kind of stuck. The teasing bothered me so bad I once took a scissors and cut out all the naps all the way up to the crown of my head." Marie Jackson started wearing her hair in a short Afro in 1968 to the chagrin of her Brooklyn neighborhood. "It was the time when everyone in my community looked at my nappy hair and was shocked," says Jackson. "Also, my church felt I needed to get a hot comb and fix my hair." For Shani Atkinson, it was her parent's commentary about her hair that wounded her the most: "My father told me that my [dred]locs looked like a pile of shit upon my head."

Black children who have naturally long and wavy hair are also targeted for teasing by their Black peers. "When I was a child, some of the [Black] kids on my block harassed me because of my hair, accusing me of thinking that I was better than them because I had 'good' hair and it was long," recalls Sheila Jenkins, a thirty-year-old graduate student in psychology. "I remember feeling hurt and rejected for something I had no control over." Veronica Williams says that for a few years during her adolescence in 1960s Philadelphia, she was afraid to go to school because she was told she had "good" hair. "There were these girls in junior high with really short hair who would follow you home from school and if they caught you they would hold you down and cut off your ponytail," remembers Williams with a shudder. Blacks are "still quibbling around skin color and hair texture," family therapist Joy DeGruy Leary says, because the psychological injuries from slavery regarding hair have not been healed. "They didn't give us the group therapy," she says, only half-joking. Not surprisingly, the affliction shows.

COLLEGE LIFE

By the time most Black teenagers make it to college, they've lived through enough difficult experiences to prepare them for a new set of challenges with their hair. One of the first things Black students have to do once they settle into campus life at a majority White institution is find a barbershop or beauty salon that caters to a Black clientele. Ruth Simmons, the former president of Smith College in Northampton, Massachusetts, has said that two of the most frequent concerns Black girls voice when considering the prestigious women's college is whether they'll be able to find a church and a Black beauty salon in close proximity to the campus. The dilemma is so pervasive that to tout their long-distance phone rates, Sprint aired a commercial about a young Black man in his new college town who would let a White barber cut his hair only if a Black barber talked him through the process over the telephone. Even though the commercial is fun and lighthearted, many teens recall the stress of being in a small town and having to travel great distances just to find an adequate beautician or barber. Some students take their chances with White beauticians who swear they know what they're doing. Cora Branson entered Mount Holyoke College in South Hadley, Massachusetts, in 1989. Fed up with traveling two and a half hours to Boston every six to eight weeks to have her relaxer touched up, she went to a salon at the local mall and asked if they knew how to work with Black hair, specifically using chemicals. "This White man said he knew what he was doing," says Branson, "so I let him. Right away I just knew it was a mistake, but he had already starting putting the relaxer on so I let him continue. He took almost half my hair out. I was angry and in pain. I just left the salon with half my hair wet, and no, I did not pay him."

To avoid the costly maintenance and annoying travel time, many Black college students become self-sufficient and do their own hair or ask other Black students for assistance. At Dartmouth College, situated in the very White hamlet of Hanover, New Hampshire, finding a professional salon that catered to a Black clientele was impossible for many years. "You could just tell that Hanover was bad for Black people's hair," says 1992 Dartmouth graduate Sheila Rogers. To compensate, once a term one of the Black sororities would hire a stylist to come up from Boston and tend to the neglected tresses of Dartmouth's Black students. The bonding that occurs between Black students facing these frustrating circumstances can be viewed as a positive by-product of attending college in a small town. Women get together to perm, braid, and style each other's hair in dormitory bathrooms, sometimes in secret but always in solidarity. Black men often seek out their "brothers" on campus to cut each other's hair. The Black students at Columbia University say that looking for a barbershop or beauty salon gives them a way to get to know the historic, culturally rich neighborhoods of Harlem and Washington Heights that border their upper Manhattan campus. "Freshman year the guys at school were so excited when they realized they'd be able to get their hair cut at the same barbershop as Malcolm X," remembers Misha Harris, a Columbia graduate.

College is also the place where Black students are forced to explain their hair-care rituals to curious and confused White roommates and dorm residents. Sarah Rubenstein is a straight-haired Jewish woman who attended college in Massachusetts. She remembers that one of the first things her first-year roommate, the daughter of a Black minister, explained to her was her hair. She washed her hair only once a week (Sundays were hair days), then blew it dry, oiled it and curled it in the morning. She applied a relaxer every two months. Once the lecture was over, there weren't supposed to be any questions, Sarah realized. "I wouldn't have felt comfortable asking them anyway," she says. "I felt very intimidated." The way Sarah remembers it, "It was like 'I'm going to tell little Whitey about my hair,' as if to say, 'You White people don't get it,'" she says. "But it's true, we don't get it."

ALL GROWN UP

Adulthood in the cycle of life with Black hair feels very similar to childhood for many men and women. There are satisfying memories of a new style or a time-honored ritual, yet there are countless interactions with a White world that doesn't understand Black hair culture. Sheila Nelson, an editor at a popular fashion magazine who straightens her hair with a hot comb, says she felt as if she was at summer camp all over again when her company retreat was themed around water activities. "According to the schedule," says Nelson, "we were supposed to go swimming and then meet for dinner like fifteen minutes later. I can't swim and then expect my hair to be presentable in fifteen minutes. If I didn't go in the water, people would think I wasn't a team player, but if I did, I knew there would be questions about why my hair didn't look the same as before." Constance Jones echoes Nelson's dilemma. A Chicago-based consultant, Jones travels a lot with her company. Once she had to share a hotel room with a White coworker, and Jones says she automatically felt herself on the defensive as well as a little self-conscious. "Here I am thirty-two years old and I'm afraid this White woman is going to think less of me because I have to put rollers in my hair at night and I use oil sheen in the morning. It's ridiculous but that's how I felt." Even though many Black people spend their childhood and college years explaining their hair-care and maintenance routines to White people, it doesn't mean the whole world was taking notes. As long as hair care remains a segregated experience in this country (salon visits, retail shopping, advertisements), Black hair culture will remain foreign.

"Unless you live with someone who is Black, as a White person you will probably remain quite ignorant of the ways in which Black hair is different from White," says Gail Jacobs, a Jewish woman who has lived with two different Black women over a period of eight years. Flipping through a mainstream magazine or watching TV or a movie, one is hard-pressed to find significant information about Black hair care, as though it were inconsequential or the same as White hair care. Jacobs says she clearly recalls witnessing Marcia Brady on *The Brady Bunch* "brushing her hair a hundred times before she went to sleep." But, Jacobs quickly counters, "I don't ever remember seeing Denise on *The Cosby Show* doing her hair in the Huxtable bathroom." As a result of this secret-society status of Black hair care in popular culture, most non-Black Americans are unable to make an educated guess about the form or function of basic Black hair tools, style techniques, or maintenance rituals. Compounding this problem is the average person's lack of knowledge regarding Black America's tangled hair history. Innocent questions always seem loaded, and curiosity can be misconstrued as mockery. "White people just want to feel [my hair] and ask stupid and annoying questions," says Anthony Riggins, now a student at Tufts

University. "That pisses me off, reminds me of my childhood, all of [those] dirty unknown fingers trying to touch my hair." Even with the best intentions, the constant questioning and uninformed commentary by White people can lead to frustration, hostility, and hurt. Some Blacks carry the burden like a heavy chip on their shoulder; others just wonder when they can stop worrying about how White America will interpret what's on top of their heads.

"When you answer the same damn question, even though it comes from five different people, you get a little tired," offers Marcia Gillespie. The most annoying queries Blacks are bombarded with range from "Why do you use grease in your hair?" to "How do you get your hair to stay like that?" One Black woman, in utter frustration over the steady stream of questions she received from her White coworkers regarding her hairstyle, started carrying around three-by-five-inch index cards with prepared answers to the most common questions she received. Undoubtedly some inquiries are indeed meant to be rude, racist, and offensive, which is why many Blacks are suspicious of so-called innocent questions. "One White guy in high school asked me why Black men have pubic hair on top of their head," recalls an angry Michele Meyerson, an Illinois native and Ph.D. candidate. "My White adviser [recently] asked me what I had been spending my time on besides my hair after I had twisted it," Meyerson adds. When you consider the fact that Black women in America already have to deal with racism and sexism, the added drama of Black hair in a White world can be interpreted as a cruel twist of fate.

There is no denying that Black hair can feel like a burden rather than a blessing. Many women harbor repressed frustrations at the time, energy, and effort Black hair requires to get it into a style society deems acceptable. "Maybe we have this envy over how easy it is for the White woman to maintain her hair," says Bernice Calvin, founder of Black Hair Expo. "Even with natural styles, we have to work at it." Everything from a day at the beach to a trip overseas requires detailed planning and serious preparation. The beach means choosing a hairstyle that won't be destroyed by a dip in the surf or finding a really cute hat. Traveling to a foreign country means packing an extra bag with emergency supplies, styling tools, and an adapter for any electrical appliances that might prove necessary. A Black female traveler can never count on finding a salon or even the most basic

Black hair products abroad. So she has to be self-sufficient—pack her own products or opt for a style like a ponytail, braids, or in a drastic move, a short natural, that requires minimal short-term maintenance. The concept of a wash-and-go style when it comes to Black hair is like pie in the sky. As Bernice Calvin intimates, Black hair is work.

"I love to hate my hair," says Vanessa Taylor. "Seriously," she continues, "I don't think I've ever been happy with my hair. A character in a movie I once saw said, 'Every day is a bad hair day for Black America.' I agree wholeheartedly." While not every Black person in America shares in Taylor's outlook, it is remarkable how many adults are in conflict. "I'm very happy with my hair, but it is a day-to-day struggle," admits Marsha Lewis, adding, "I hate the way our hair can speak so many words for us before we open our mouths." One thirty-five-year-old Black woman who grew up in the Midwest says that she has only recently moved from a love/hate relationship with her hair to one of acceptance. "For years I pushed, pounded, fried, dyed, refried, laid down, crocheted, braided, extended, Luster Curled, Jheri Curled, blow-dried, hot-combed, curling-ironed, hair-rollered [my hair] trying to get it to make sense to the rest of the world. I wanted long, flowing tresses just like Barbie and Diana Ross," she says. If she only knew: Barbie's hair is plastic, and Ms. Ross wears a weave.

It would be erroneous to assume that all Black people dislike their hair or even have problems working with it. From celebrity stylists to adolescent boys on the road to self-discovery, Black people often use their hair as a medium for celebrating creative energy. "I love my hair," says Penn State student Lois Baxter. "I wake up every day and wonder how I was able to grow [dred]locs on my head. I love to touch my hair and I love to take care of her." The texture of Black hair, in its natural form or chemically altered, is also conducive to a plethora of styling options. "Kinky hair . . . relaxes and straightens easily, and can hold curly styles with great success," writes New York–based celebrity stylist Kevin Mancuso in his book *The Mane Thing.* "Kinky hair is also self-supportive," Mancuso writes. "What this means is that in its naturally dry state, it can be fashioned into shapes . . . and hold the style with relative ease and not need spraying." Curls, finger waves, braids, twists—the list of styling variations is endless. Black people can change their hairstyle to match their mood and satisfy their every whim. "I like to find new, unique things to do with my hair," says Habiba

Anan, a Washington, D.C., native. "Before it was through the use of a combination of colors. Now it's more in terms of styles. I feel like I'm often defending my hair because it's not straight and slick, [but] I just laugh because I couldn't be happier with it."

The Beauty Parlor and Barbershop: Sanctified Space

Whether Black people view their hair as crowning glory or lifelong frustration, finding the right person to clip it, cut it, and style it is tantamount to selecting a godparent for one's child. It is precious material to hand over to a stranger. For many men and women the relationship with their hairstylist lasts longer than some marriages. Wesleyan graduate Tabitha Brown wrote her college entrance essay on the person who had the most influence on her life: her hairdresser. "My hairdresser was so influential because each phase of my school-age life was marked by a different hairstyle—from a stacked asymmetrical Philly cut, to dredlocs—and my hairdresser in that sense was like the navigator of my social circumstance." Finding just the right beauty salon or barbershop is equally important.

Black salons in urban meccas like New York, Los Angeles, and Detroit are known for staying open to the wee hours of the night and sometimes twenty-four hours to accommodate customers who crave intricate braided styles that may require as much as eight to ten hours to achieve or for those who just can't make it during nine-to-five business hours. Some women are so self-conscious, so unwilling to let people see them even for one day without their hair styled, that when it's time for a new 'do, they make midnight appointments to ensure a perfect coiffure by the time the rest of the world is rising.

Some people would argue that the distinction between Black and White hair salons and barbershops is not so great in terms of physical design or even social importance—both serve as a site of community and aesthetic interaction. Midge Wilson and Kathy Russell, coauthors of *Divided Sisters: Bridging the Gap Between Black Women and White Women*, think otherwise. "Trips to the beauty parlor for most White women are primarily functional," they write. "In contrast, when African-American women go to the beauty parlor—and this was especially true when so many more were 'hot combing'—there is a lot of time to share problems with others." In her essay "The Art of the Ponytail," gen-x writer Akkida McDowell remembers her childhood beauty parlor visits this way:

> I saw women handling real business against a backdrop of music, gossip, steam and oil sheen. I encountered professional women, housewives, teachers and women from other walks of life. . . . I discovered the latest news, saw the recent fashion trends, ate delicious, home-cooked food and heard grown folks' talk. . . . I enjoyed this nurturing ritual and scarcely noted the tugging and twisting. I bonded with my grandmother and my mother and flourished in the company of the women in the shop.

The camaraderie women experience at the salon also occurs at the barbershop among Black men. Leroy Carter, thirty-three, grew up in Nashville, Tennessee, and reminisces about the good old days: "One of the most satisfying times in my life was going to the barbershop and getting a clear-cut fade on Saturday mornings, bonding with other brothers, talking

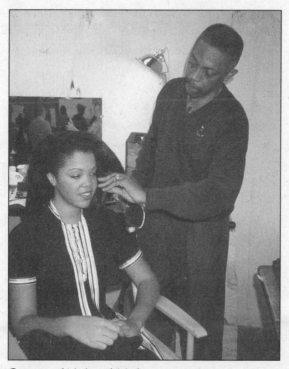

Courtesy of Nathaniel Mathis.

I'se in Town, Honey:
The Life of Aunt Jemima

A symbol since 1889, the logo of Aunt Jemima and her lesser-known sister, Mrs. Butterworth, made the Mammy an image that was as common and comfortable as a warm breakfast of pancakes and syrup. The trademark, of a fat, happy Black woman in an apron and kerchief, was the first in American history to be personified, and by 1990 there were forty products featuring the smiling Black woman. Sales of these goods totalled three hundred million dollars annually. Following is the sordid tale of race, sex, and hair that accompanied the good aunt's history.

1889: Chris L. Rutt and Charles G. Underwood create the first ready-made pancake mix. They embark on a search for a marketing logo to help reassure White American housewives that the newfangled idea of an "instant" food mix is a good thing. The search takes them to a Missouri vaudeville house. Blackface minstrel comedians Baker and Farrell bring the house down with a popular tune of the day, "Aunt Jemima." Dressed in aprons and red bandannas, Baker and Farrell had hit on exactly what Rutt was searching for to sell his pancakes—the Black just-there-to-please-the-White-folks Mammy of antebellum plantation days. Rutt borrows one more thing from the minstrel act—the crudely drawn sketch of a Black Mammy that appeared on the vaudeville duo's posters.

1893: New company owner R. T. Davis goes on a national search for a real woman to be Aunt Jemima. He finds Kentucky ex-slave Nancy Green. The logo is changed to look like her. Green's debut is at the 1893 World's Columbian Exposition in Chicago. Green stands next to a twenty-four-foot-high flour barrel and cooks pancakes, sings songs, and tells stories of the Old South to interested passersby. Souvenir buttons are distributed featuring the Aunt Jemima image and the slogan "I'se in Town, Honey." Fifty thousand orders for pancake mix are placed by the end of the fair. "I'se in Town, Honey" becomes the slogan for billboards placed in cities around the United States. A free pamphlet is published called "The Life of Aunt Jemima, the Most Famous Colored Woman in the World." Green begins a string of appearances at fairs, food shows, grocery stores, and festivals. She would portray Aunt Jemima until her death in 1923.

1896: The R. T. Davis Mills Company introduces customers to the entire Aunt Jemima family, a line of rag dolls featuring the familiar kerchiefed woman and her Uncle Mose and two moppets, Diana and Wade. For four cents (the cost of stamps) one can receive "The Life History of Aunt Jemima and Her Pickaninny Dolls." It's a hit.

1926: The rag dolls were such a hit that the R. T. Davis Mills Company decides to offer them again. Through an advertisement that runs in the leading White women's magazine *Ladies Home Journal,* the dolls are scooped up by women who say that they were raised with the dolls and can't wait to get one for their daughters. That same year, the Quaker Oats Company purchases the R. T. Davis Mills Company.

1933: Anna Robinson becomes the second Aunt Jemima. She weighs in at 350 pounds and is sent around the nation to pose with celebrities, dignitaries, and politicians at nightclubs and various hot spots. The logo is redesigned using her likeness, and Aunt Jemima becomes heavier and darker-skinned.

1948: Edith Wharton becomes the next living, breathing Aunt Jemima. She appears on radio, television, and in personal appearances throughout the U.S. It was Wharton's likeness that was to appear on the logo through the 1980s.

Late 1950s: The Aunt Jemima product line, featuring salt and pepper shakers, cookie jars, a pottery set of condiment holders, and various cardboard items, is discontinued. Black consumers, empowered by the Civil Rights movement, used their economic leverage to show Quaker Oats that they saw the images as virulent.

1957: Aylene Lewis takes over as Aunt Jemima. While her image never makes the front of any syrup bottles, Lewis gains popularity by serving pancakes at the Aunt Jemima Kitchen Restaurant in Disneyland. Lewis dishes up breakfast in a bandanna, matching skirt, and a shawl. Some of her famous customers are Walt Disney and Benny Goodman.

1968: At the height of the Black Power movement, African-Americans threaten to boycott Quaker Oats if something isn't done about Aunt Jemima. The first thing to go is the headscarf, replaced by a headband. In order to get more distance from the fat Black Mammy stereotype, Quaker Oats eventually also drastically reduces Aunt Jemima's weight and makes her appear much younger.

July 1989: Aunt Jemima's headband is replaced with a permed, gray-streaked hairstyle. She is also given pearl earrings and a lace collar. Some comment that she looks like a Black Betty Crocker. Quaker Oats says that the new look is meant to "present Aunt Jemima in a more contemporary light, while preserving the important attributes of warmth, quality, good taste, heritage, and reliability." Although there were no Black women with perms and pearls serving breakfast to Whites in America's heritage, Quaker Oats's latest update at least cuts back on the most offensive elements of the image. Her "reassuring" smile stays the same.

about everything and nothing in particular." Some men are so loyal to their barber that they will drive miles out of their way to receive his services. Cecil Brown, fifty-five, says he was on a quest to find the perfect barber for over thirty-one years. When he discovered the wildly popular urban-chic Philadelphia Hair Company in that city's Germantown section five years ago, he stopped looking. Even though Brown lives almost an hour away and may have to wait several hours on Saturdays before his favorite barber can fit him in, he says it's worth the effort. "It's the way I treat him and the service we provide," says Brown's barber, Dennis Scanton. The Philadelphia Hair Company is the type of establishment where Black men go to get pampered, watch the game, and while away an entire Saturday afternoon in good company. "You get a haircut *here*, it's like entertainment," promises Scanton.

Social Organization

THE BEAUTY MYTHS

Black or White, male or female, the quest to be beautiful has a lot to do with attracting someone of the opposite sex, and worldwide, hair plays an important role in determining beauty. Since the beauty standards in this country are set according to a White aesthetic—from Miss America to the Barbie doll—Black women are left with precious few places to turn to find an image of beauty that showcases unstraightened tresses and natural hairstyles. "We are an appearance-obsessed culture and our obsession with looks is critical to the maintenance of sexism and racism," opines bell hooks. On the one hand, hooks says, "White women have lots of issues about their hair, but they also have lots of affirmation for their hair. [Black people] don't have the overall cultural affirmation that counters the negative obsession." Tracey Moore, a graduate student in California, struggles with this issue. "I go from bouts of adoration for my hair to disdain. . . . The moment I get up and see that I have to fix my hair, I just wish that I had straight black hair that fell easily into place without the pulling and brushing."

Even though women are often more vocal about their desire for straight hair, Black men are a fundamental part of the equation. Since Black males are raised in the same environments as females, it is inevitable that many of them will find straight hair desirable for women and sometimes for themselves. Jack Thompson had a Black mother and a White father and was told, growing up in 1980s Kansas City, that thanks to his dad he had "a good head of hair." Still, Thompson wanted perfectly straight hair like his father and begged his mother to take him to the barbershop and straighten his hair. "I wanted to be like my father," recalls Thompson. "I wanted to be White." Thompson says his mother agreed and took him to the barbershop on a Saturday afternoon when the shop was full of Black men. "She walks me into the shop, stands me in the middle of the room, and says [to the barber], 'He wants to get his hair pressed straight so he can be White like his daddy, so I'll leave him here with you to take care of it,'" says Thompson. "The room exploded. By the time I got into the chair, I just wanted a trim." Not surprisingly, this quest for straight hair is essentially new wording for desiring "good" hair. In an essay published in her 1992 *Black Looks* collection, bell hooks examines this continued obsession: "Despite civil rights struggle, the 1960s' black power movement, and the power of slogans like 'Black is beautiful,' masses of black people continue to be socialized via mass media and non-progressive educational systems to internalize white supremacist thoughts and values."

In this country, it is impossible to ignore the fact that pop culture paradigms of beautiful Black women are coiffed with long, straight hair. When Mattel introduced its first Black Barbie doll in 1980, she had long, loosely curled hair. Ten years later when the toy company updated its brown-skinned mannequins in an effort to make them appear more ethnic, Black Barbie—recast as Shani—still managed to keep her long, flowing mane. "To be truly realistic, one [Shani doll] should have shorter hair, but little girls of all races love hair play," said a Mattel executive. "We added more texture, but we can't change the fact that long, combable hair is still a key seller."

The transition from Barbie dolls to living dolls leads to Tyra Banks and Naomi Campbell, two of the best-known Black supermodels. These two international celebrities are hardly ever showcased without a cascading weave falling down their backs. From movie stars to video extras, Black women in the entertainment industry are expected to approximate a White standard of beauty. "The images we are given in the media that are associated with status are consistent with Eurocentric images," Michael L. Blakely, a physical anthropologist at Howard University, told *Essence* magazine. "There seems to be less appreciation for the aesthetic value of tropical African biology," he added. Talent agent and former model Bethann Hardison explained to *Essence* in 1991 why White fashion directors and advertising executives tend to favor Black women with light skin and long hair. "It's natural," Hardison said. "They want a girl who looks like them. Their whole nation is thinking about themselves. They are not thinking about Black people."

Among the popular Black actresses and models of the late eighties and nineties, there was one major exception to the long-haired ideal—a Black model named Roshumba. This dark-skinned woman wore her hair in a short natural cut. As unusual as her success as a short-haired model was, it was even more notable because she was a dark-skinned, short-haired African-American model, an image that seemed to disregard all the tenets of a Eurocentric beauty ideal. In an early 1990s *Essence* article she recalled

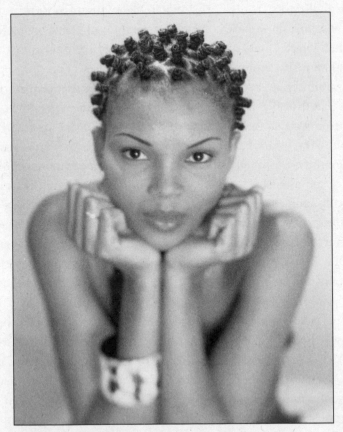

Nubian knots. © Hosea L. Johnson.

an experience with a photographer: "I got booked for an ad and they told me to bring some wigs. I showed up without them and told the photographer, 'Either shoot me with my own 'fro or we don't do it.'" As revolutionary as Roshumba's success may have seemed, her "rebel stance" was undercut by the fact that in the majority of articles written about her, the emphasis was on what an exception she was. Instead of her look opening doors for more short-haired Black models, she remained an anomaly.

COURTSHIP

Bombardment by images of Black females with long hair, coupled with historical condemnation of short natural hair, plays a great role in the mating rituals between Black men and women. Many Black women believe that to be attractive to men, they have to have long, straight hair. "I didn't cut my hair short prior to 1999 because my boyfriend kept reminding me how much better I would look with long hair," says Monisha Lincoln. "Although I love the easy care and upkeep, I feel infinitely less sexy and womanly with short hair."

Some woman feel compelled to add on fake hair to get the length and texture Black men will respond to, based on the images celebrated in popular culture, both White and Black. "The proliferation . . . of hair weaves and braided extensions is a manifestation of Black women's desire for hair that is not only straight but long, the better to toss," writes author and journalist Jill Nelson. "To Black women, the message sent by the culture of beauty remains the same, i.e., that we genetically lack a fundamental element of desirability." Wearing hair weaves and extensions, then, for many women, seems part of the required accessorizing process to snag a male partner, Black or White.

Ironically, Black men consistently go on record saying they would much rather see a woman's real hair than something fake. In a 1991 *Essence* article examining the debate, Black men strongly voiced their opinions against the add-on hair game, saying they'd never want to be with a woman who wore a weave or extensions. "Work with what you have," pleaded one man who was tired of seeing women with weaves. Second-year college student Willie Johnson says he'd never date a girl with a weave. He says, "I really like long hair, but if it came out or disappeared one day and came back the next, I ain't down with that." Journalist Jerry Rogers takes it one step further: "I think natural hair is the sexist thing on a Black woman. I just think the feel of a Black woman's hair in one's hands is perfectly wonderful."

While championing short natural hair may seem the culturally correct thing to do, many Black women say that reality is a different story. "When I'm intimate with [Black] men, they don't want to touch my hair," says Charline Cannon, a marketing manager in the California Bay Area who keeps her hair in a short natural. "But Black women I know with long permed hair say their men can't wait to touch it. Maybe guys think that touching a Black women's hair with a natural would be like touching a man's head," Cannon theorizes. When Jill Nelson shaved off most of her hair in 1996 she wrote in her autobiography, "Most Black men's eyes skip over me rapidly, distastefully, as if they do not care to see someone who looks like me."

By the early 1990s, Black hair-care manufacturers were strongly reinforcing the idea that Black men prefer straight hair, by creating most of their advertisements for straightening products—especially relaxers—with the suggestion that straight hair was the key to a Black man's heart. "Look at Him! He Can't Keep His Eyes Off My Hair!" screamed a TCB Bone Strait relaxer ad. Clearly every Black man cannot be lumped into a single category when it comes to personal preferences for a woman's hair, but the media, entertainment industry, and advertisers continue to perpetuate the myth that straight, long hair equals beauty.

THE HAIR HIERARCHY

Straight hair versus kinky. Long hair versus short. The social order of Black hair culture has a place for every hair type. Once upon a time the categories were simple: a person either had "good" or "bad" hair. After emancipation, straight hair implied education and modernity, and braided styles covered with a head rag branded one countrified and backward. The Afro instituted a new consciousness and turned the pecking order on its head as hair became political. Today, with the variety of styles available, the margin for error is great, but Black people tend to assume that certain styles say something about a person's socioeconomic status. Kathy Y. Russell, Midge Wilson, and Ronald Hall, authors of the book *The Color Complex*, assert the following hypothesis:

All things being equal, a Black woman whose hair grows naturally straight is usually thought to be from a 'better' family than a woman whose hair is nappy. Black women who wear natural styles cut across socioeconomic lines, but a politically defiant style like dredlocs is generally a middle-class expression of Black consciousness. Poor Black women with very kinky hair strive instead for straighter-looking hair. . . .

Author and cultural historian Harriette Cole hesitates to confirm that certain hairstyles correlate with class or social status, but she does admit that Black women who tend to wear "black-tie hair at all times of the day, often unnaturally colored and frozen in place" are going to be looked at as lower-class. Although it sounds like some sort of intraracial discrimination, judging people by their hairstyle is a common practice in American culture. It is one way Americans compartmentalize and categorize the people they encounter. When a White woman wears a lot of makeup and a hairstyle that requires an entire can of aerosol hair spray to maintain, people may make assumptions about her class background. Likewise Mary Lewis, an African-American loan officer in Wisconsin, finds herself making economic assumptions about Black women who wear weaves. "A lot of times you see weaves on Black women who are lower income and single," Lewis explains. "They feel that wearing a weave will help them get a boyfriend, when in fact most men don't care for them. But it's not just the hair, it's the acrylic nails, the gold teeth with the star, and all that awful makeup." Of course different styles—for men and women—take on different meanings depending on what part of the country a person visits. "My husband has shoulder-length dredlocs," says Jessica Dugger, a graduate student in North Carolina, "and in different parts of the country he has been looked upon as a scholar, a rap/movie star, an activist, a bum, or a drug dealer." Black men who wear natural styles like Afros, cornrows, or braids are often viewed as thuglike, while a Black man with relaxed or processed hair might be associated with shady nightclub dealings and a pimp-friendly lifestyle.

If it is hard to believe that hair can be so telling about a person's socioeconomic background, consider Aunt Jemima. In 1989 when Quaker Oats, Aunt Jemima's parent company, wanted to upgrade Auntie J. from house servant to middle-class grandmother, they simply unwrapped her hair from its signature red kerchief and apparently gave her a relaxer—all nice, new, and loosely curled. Aunt Jemima's new style made it look as if America's favorite Mammy had stepped out of the kitchen and into the suburbs.

Battling the Forces of Evil

In seventh-grade social studies class, children are taught about nation building. One of the common techniques to fuel a country's nationalistic fervor is to go to war against a common enemy. It is no different within the culture of Black hair. Black people meeting for the first time can be fast friends in a matter of moments when together they face off against the enemy—at the beach, the beauty parlor, or boarding school.

Water

Within the culture of Black hair, water is the enduring enemy. Parents often admonish their kids to take care that nothing happens to make their hair get messy or "turn back." "Nothing" usually implies coming into contact with moisture (i.e., rain, sweat, or a swimming pool). Although the drastic examples of Black people drowning because they never learned to swim for fear of ruining their hairstyle have been relegated to folklore, most Black women can still remember the bittersweet pull of a swimming pool or a lake in the heat of summer. They wanted to jump in with the rest of the kids but were afraid of how their mother might react if she saw that the once perfect hairstyle had been destroyed—not to mention the horrid thought of having to sit through another session of pulling and tugging the kinks out. A little Black girl always has to ask herself "Is it worth it?" And then, of course, if the swimming session includes White folks, there is always a sense of insecurity over how "those people" will react when the hair reverts back to its naturally puffy condition. "When I was younger I would feel self-conscious when I went swimming with my White friends," says Tasha Jones. My hair didn't look the same as theirs when it dried and I felt like an outsider because of it."

Many Black women can sympathize with Tasha's feelings, having been in the same situation themselves at one time or another. And it doesn't get better with age. For some Black women it gets worse, as it begins to seem impossible to attract the opposite sex with hair that looks "puffy" and "frizzy" at the beach or poolside—not to mention the headache of having to go home and comb through the tangles, blow-dry, and restyle. "I've been to pool parties," says Janice Michaels, "where girls don't even get in for fear they would ruin their hair." The bad jokes about Black people not being able to swim regrettably gain credence from the multitudes of Black women who refuse to take the plunge, staunchly protecting their hair. On the other hand, some Black women are like Sienna Jacobs, who has naturally long, wavy hair and met most of her boyfriends at pool parties because her hair stayed straight even when wet. "Once everyone got wet, here I was with all this wavy hair down to my butt," says Jacobs. "I looked like those White models in beach shots. . . . I know men noticed me because of it." Even though Jacobs received a lot of male attention because of her flowing locs, she also received the scathing glares of many a Black female shackled to the sidelines trying to keep her hair high and dry.

CHEMICALS

Some members of the Black hair-care establishment would argue that the real enemy of their crowning glory is not water but chemicals, specifically chemical relaxers. Wearing a relaxer means being at the mercy of one's hair. "Perms are really like jail," laments twenty-seven-year-old opera singer Karyn Hall, who has worn her hair relaxed since the age of five. "You are totally locked into this cycle with them, and they restrict so much of what you can do—swimming, pool parties, going out in the rain."

Since there are plenty of Black men and women happily relaxing their hair, the chemicals-as-jail opinion is not unanimous. Juanita James views her monthly relaxer appointment as nothing more than a means to an end. "I always had this idea that getting my hair straightened allowed my hair to be combed without my mother tearing my brains out," says James, who has been chemically relaxing her hair for the past twenty years. "I thought of [it] as a mechanism to make your hair combable." Harriette Cole, who wears her hair in a short, stylish natural, agrees that relaxed hair is easy to manage if properly cared for, but therein lies a more sinister problem. "It takes care and attention and time to handle natural hair," Cole explains. "Something we have lost from our African culture are the rituals of health and beauty and taking time to anoint ourselves. And the first way we lost it was in our hair."

Many Black people go through life never knowing the style and beauty options natural hair offers. With over 60 percent of Black American women wearing their hair relaxed and an estimated 5 percent using a hot comb to straighten it, there are precious few natural-hair role models out there for visual consumption. Outside major cities like Chicago, New York, and Los Angeles, a Black person is hard-pressed even to find a Black stylist who knows how to work with natural hair. "For so long, something as simple as keeping their hair natural was a problem for a lot of women," former model Peggy Dillard told *Essence* magazine about her inspiration to open a beauty salon specializing in natural hair. "If they had gone to any Black salon in New York City, at some point someone might have said, 'Why don't you straighten your hair?' or cut it off if they have locs. I thought they deserved a better choice and some support." Dillard opened Turning Heads salon in Harlem in 1986.

Lonnice Brittenum Bonner, a professed former slave to chemicals, self-published a book, *Good Hair: For Colored Girls Who've Considered Weaves When the Chemicals Became Too Ruff,* in 1994 because she recognized the ignorance of most Black women regarding their own hair. Dozens of Black women responded to this how-to-deal-with-natural-hair tome with praise and gratitude, admitting they never knew there was an alternative to straight hair. One reader from Massachusetts gushed that Bonner "teaches you how to work with Black hair rather than against it. She lets us know something we should have known all along: the rules for White women's hair don't apply to ours."

For many women the experience of cutting off their relaxed hair for the first time and feeling the texture of their natural hair is like an epiphany. Says Cynthia Mason, "I slowly came to the conclusion that I didn't need long, straight hair to be beautiful. With shoulder-length hair I went to Turning Heads in Harlem and got my hair cut into a short natural Afro. I thought I would cry, but I was beaming and revitalized."

THE OTHER

Since Black people themselves admittedly don't know everything about their own natural hair, it hardly seems fair to hold White people up to similar expectations. However, White people's lack of knowledge about Black hair can be a dangerous deficiency in some cases. Jackie Taylor, thirty-nine, relates the following experience:

> I was a kid in an orphanage facility. Some White women were in charge of getting the kids ready for bed. They believed, as many White women do, in brushing or combing the hair before bed. These women had washed my hair before my bedtime and were combing it out with such force I thought they were going to tear my head off. I cried so hard from the pain. By the time they were done, I felt that I had suffered a concussion by my brain being banged around in my skull and from all the pulling and conking upside the head.

White people's misconceptions and misinformation regarding Black hair are well known in the Black community. This is a real concern that has actually influenced national policies regarding interracial adoptions. The National Association of Black Social Workers, as late as 1999, defended its position against interracial adoptions (namely, White couples adopting Black children) by citing hair issues as a legitimate concern. "In a nutshell, African-Americans are in the best position to teach African-American children how to survive in this country as African-Americans," Rudolph C. Smith, president of the association told the Denver *Rocky Mountain News*. "White females can't teach young Black girls how to comb their hair; White men can't teach young Black boys what to do on the street when the cops stop you." Though they would be loath to agree with Smith's analysis, many White women who have half-Black children admit that tackling a head of nappy hair is often a daunting experience. Kobe Winston, a 1995 alumna of Kenyon College in Ohio, witnessed the results of that challenge firsthand. "There was this one girl on campus, Hope, and we used to always wonder why her hair was such a mess," recalls Winston. Winston and her Black girlfriends later found out that Hope had been raised by her White mother in Vermont. "She didn't know what a hot comb was. She didn't understand the concept of a blow-dryer with a comb attachment. She did her hair like she was White. She would just wash her hair every day and leave it," Winston says incredulously. Finally, a Black student took Hope aside, broached the subject of hair, and taught her the tricks of the trade. She was grateful and said she hadn't realized there was a different way to care for Black hair. In a happy endnote, Winston says she recently ran into Hope and her hair looked "really nice."

Knowledge of Culture

The roots of Black hair culture emerged from the Black experience in America and are not just a by-product of having tight, kinky coils resting on the head. African women living in this country, for example, are often overwhelmed by all the drama tangled up in the hair. "In Nigeria you can wear a weave or a wig and it's not an issue," declares Ifoema Ibo, a graphic designer living in New York. "In Africa the hair is purely to decorate. It's different here because of the race issue. If you straighten your hair here you want to be White." Njeri Waiganjo, a native Kenyan who came to the United States to attend college, agrees with Ibo and adds, "What was a surprise to me was [that] the way you do your hair can be a political statement. I had never seen that." Black or White, the transmission of Black hair culture comes only from living the life. Like any other culture it is learned and shared within the community from which it sprang. Lisa Jones, screenwriter and columnist, said it best: "Everything I know about American history I learned from looking at Black people's hair. It's the perfect metaphor for the African experiment here: the toll of slavery and the costs of remaining. It's all in the hair."

7

Hair Today,
Hair Tomorrow:
1995–2000

Nathaniel Mathis never expected to be immortalized. The Washington, D.C., barber was content just to nurse his clients' hair to good health. Over the years, however, through a combination of marketing chutzpah and a real talent with hair, he advanced from local barber to Hollywood image consultant. He's been called the Mahatma of Hair by *Time* magazine but he will always be known as the Bush Doctor. At the end of the twentieth century, Mathis, sixty-three, acquired his latest accolade: first African-American hairdresser to be honored by the Smithsonian Institution's National Museum of American History. The Nathaniel Mathis Collection of Barbering and Beauty Culture, currently housed in the museum's archives, bears witness to Mathis's extraordinary thirty-six-year career in the world of Black hair. Some of the standout moments include his 1976 participation in the World Hair Olympics (the first African-American to do so); his 1983 tour of West Africa, where he received the royal treatment for introducing African women to the curly perm; and most recently his turn as stylist to the stars on the sets of big-screen movies like *Dick* and *Liberty Heights*. "We turn down many more collections than we can accept," noted Smithsonian Chief Archivist John Fleckner. "We've inherited a long visual heritage, and some of it's full of stereotypes. It's great to be able to include some of the images Black people have made of themselves." Mathis's personal artifacts, tools, trophies, and his patented multipocketed barber's vest are now all available for public appreciation.

The fact that an American institution as august as the Smithsonian would recognize a humble man for his contributions to beauty culture says a lot about Nat Mathis, but it says even more about Black hair. At the dawn of the

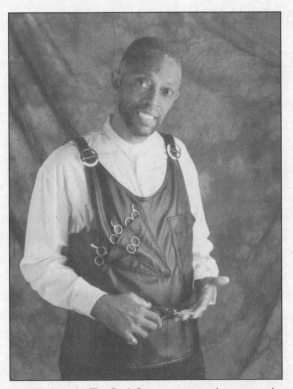

Nat Mathis, aka The Bush Doctor, wearing his patented barber's apron. Courtesy of Nathaniel Mathis.

twenty-first century, the image makers and power brokers in American culture are finally recognizing the influence Black hair has had in shaping American culture. Black hair has also been deemed important enough for serious scholarship. In the last decade of the twentieth century, classes dedicated exclusively to the history and politics of Black hair were taught at America's most esteemed institutions of higher learning, such as Stanford University. Scholars and historians—both Black and White—were dedicating research time and money to serious investigations into Black hair culture. At the 1999 convention of the American Association of Anthropologists, held in Chicago, there were at least half a dozen presentations made on different aspects of Black hair, including the politics of hair among African-American women, the political economy of hair weaving, and the business culture surrounding Annie Turnbo Malone's Poro Products company. To usher in the new century, in February 2000, the Museum for African Art in New York City launched a two-year traveling exhibition dedicated entirely to Black hair. The *Hair in African Art and Culture* exhibit examined the significance of hair in Africa and explored the cross-cultural relationship between African and African-American hair. By the looks of things, Black hair has finally earned its due.

But of course change is a gradual process, and progress comes at a price. Over three hundred years of a tangled and often painful history cannot be washed away with a museum exhibit and goodwill. Black people still grapple with a feeling of otherness when it comes to their hair, and White people remain unaware of the need for healing. Employing a modified theory of physics, for every positive action that occurs in the realm of Black hair (like the celebration of the Bush Doctor), there is an equal and opposite negative action experienced by any number of young Black girls who are shamed into believing their hair is ugly if it isn't straight and long. As we enter the twenty-first century it is important to look at both the good and the bad when we try to ascertain just how far we've come in untangling the roots of Black hair in America.

Outside the hallowed halls of academia, talk about Black hair has shifted away from the political arena and into the realm of fashion and style. Black women are going blond because they want to, Black teenage boys are wearing cornrows and Afros in emulation of rappers and athletes, and Tyra Banks can appear on *Oprah* and tell the whole world she wears a weave without fear of ostracism or complaints that she is trying to be White. Accusations about cultural misappropriation have dissolved into conversations about sharing. White people and Asians are getting their hair braided in African-inspired styles in record numbers. Upscale beauty salons in New York and California have developed something called a "Rasta perm"—a chemical formula for turning straight White or Asian hair into something that approximates dredlocs in mere minutes—and for only two hundred dollars a pop. Droves of non-Black women in Hollywood (and across the nation) have latched onto the extensions and hairpiece craze. Gwyneth Paltrow wore extensions to the

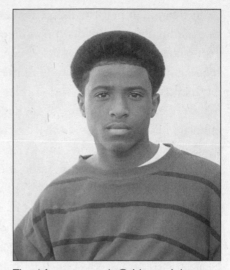

The Afro reinvented. © Hosea Johnson.

1998 Academy Awards, as did Jennifer Love Hewitt when she was named *Cosmopolitan*'s Fun Fearless Female of 2000. As Ms. Oprah Winfrey herself said on her show late in 1999, "Even the White people know what weaves are. That means they're here to stay." "The bottom line is it's just about style," offers *Ms.* magazine's Marcia Gillespie, who wears her salt-and-pepper natural hair in glorious little twists. "We have to realize that cultural stuff is being borrowed and transformed, copied, imitated, and shared back and forth. That's part of the process of being on this planet." Image consultant and author Harriette Cole views this as more like cosmic recompense. "I don't know if I would call it 'divine revenge,' but definitely the 'divine twist.' All of these people are adopting our hairstyles, and I'm sure most of it is not even conscious."

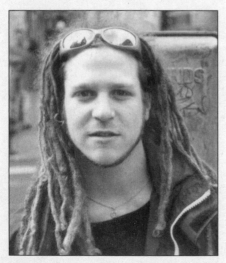

White men do wear dreds. © Alfonso Smith.

With this anything-goes atmosphere, Black men and women are finally freer than ever before to chose a hairstyle based on personal taste rather than what mainstream society deems acceptable. Nelson Boyce is the advertising sales director for a major pop culture magazine in New York City. Even though he handles many of the more conservative corporate accounts, he decided to grow dredlocs regardless of the friction it might cause. "I felt my professionalism would stand out beyond my hair," the 1991 Harvard graduate states with conviction. "Once people heard what I had to say, I figured [my hair] would be a nonfactor." To date, Boyce has not received a single complaint about his hair from his superiors or from the White clients to whom he sells advertising space.

When African-American journalist Farai Chideya was offered an on-air correspondent position with ABC news in 1997, the then twenty-seven-year-old brought up the hair thing right away. "I told them I was not going to change my hair," says Chideya. ABC brass didn't balk, and Chideya was allowed to keep her silky dred hairstyle (a style that approximates dredlocs wrapped with synthetic silk). "It was pretty much a nonissue," Chideya says, "but I just felt I had to bring it up." With role models like the dredloced entertainers Lauryn Hill and Lisa Bonet, the headwrapped singer-actress Erykah Badu, and Afro wild-child musician Lenny Kravitz (formerly a dred wearer), Blacks and Whites have alternative visual images to the straight versus nappy historical references.

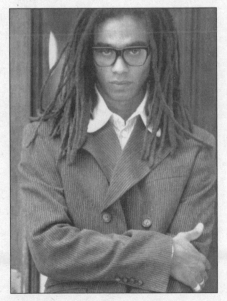

When it comes to hair today, says actress Lisa Bonet, "anything goes as far as expressing yourself and feeling beautiful and happy."

White America, in fact, has become so comfortable with formerly rebellious Black hairstyles that they've co-opted them for their own use. Corporate giant IBM strays from the pack by using a Black model sporting short natural twists in the advertisements showcasing its Internet presence. Fashion houses like John Galliano and Chanel are wont to outfit their skinny White models in dredloc styles and multicolored

Dreds go to work. © Alfonso Smith.

Afro wigs for the Paris runway shows to create a buzz. Middle America clothing stores like Banana Republic, The Gap, and J. Crew are now featuring Black models in their ads with brilliant natural hairstyles. In a 1999 Levi's Jeans ad, a Black man wearing dredlocs holds a sign that reads "Conformity leads to mediocrity."

Change is also occurring within the Black community, as more and more people embrace natural styles that emphasize the unique texture of Black hair rather than trying to hide it. With the proliferation of magazines like *Braids and Beauty,* launched in 1994, whose editorial content is dedicated to natural hairstyles, there are convenient, affordable resources more readily available to educate people about chemical alternatives.

This is not to say that all of Black America is scurrying to "free up" their roots. Quite the contrary. When trendsetters like hip-hop queens Lil' Kim and Mary J. Blige change their hair color to match their mood and outfits, and their legions of fans follow suit, there is nothing natural going on there. And what should be made of the striking Black woman in the Dark & Lovely hair color ad who sports dredlocs, but they are dyed blond? The point is that more and more Black people are letting go of the pain, the drama, and community policing over hair and adopting a more open-minded mentality. Television producer Yvette Bowser Lee obviously noted the trend when she created the character of Regine (played by Kim Fields) in 1993 for her Fox sitcom *Living Single.* In every episode Regine sported several different wigs, weaves, and hairpieces and did not try to pass them off as her real hair. Sometimes she even took them off on-camera. For Regine, hair was just an accessory. When it comes to the Black hair game, opines Bernice Calvin, "I think we've all calmed down."

Where there used to be embarrassment and secrecy about Black hair, now there is a growing sense of openness and honesty. Supermodel Tyra Banks appeared on *Oprah* in November 1999 and quite bluntly admitted her hair was fake. Why? Because the down-to-earth model knows how unrealistic and dangerous it is for people to aspire to unnatural beauty standards. Says Banks, "Many celebrities have images that are larger than life [and] this can be very intimidating to the public, particularly young women. It's important for me to be honest about the tricks I use." One of Tyra's tricks: "Personally, I don't color my hair at all. I use clip-in highlights. This allows for quick and easy changes and keeps my hair healthy." Toni Braxton, the former pixie cut queen, is equally candid about her hair habits. "If you ever see my hair really long, like past my shoulders," the R&B diva told *Essence* magazine, "girl, it's a weave—don't ever think anything else."

Celebrate Good Times

As Black hair history and culture began to push their way into mainstream consciousness, the art world began to take notice. British artist Chris Ofili, the infamous creator of the elephant dung–enhanced Madonna and Child painting that made international headlines in 1999, is equally famous for his series of "Afrodizzia" paintings that celebrate the Afro's form, fame, and history. Like the Madonna painting, his Afro-inspired works are multimedia creations sprinkled with animal feces, but they also feature famous Black people who made the Afro legendary. Ofili has received international acclaim for the paintings, critics praising the series as "inspired" and "thought provoking." Meanwhile, documentary filmmakers are exploring everything from the history of Black hair to the hair's artistic expression. Philadelphia-based hairstylist Yvette Smalls, who counts songstress Erykah Badu and poet Sonia Sanchez as clients, explored the historical and cultural meaning of Black hair in a forty-minute documentary titled *Hair Stories*. Nigerian-born Andrew Dosumnu, on the other hand, checked out the outrageousness of the internationally renowned styling competition Hair Wars in his forty-five-minute documentary *Hot Irons*. Dosumnu's poignant but ultimately hilarious peek into the fierce competitiveness of the show illustrated the creative energy Black people display when it comes to hair. The true testament to the success of *Hot Irons* is that it has not been confined solely to African-American audiences. The movie played in art-house theaters around the world and received awards and critical praise from film critics and social scientists alike.

By the final years of the 1990s it looked as if Black hair was safe for Black people to talk about, and appropriate for White people to champion. A case in point is the arresting picture book *Dreads*. Written by two Italian men in 1999, the book is a photographic exploration of what dredlocs mean to different people around the globe. Whites and Blacks and everyone in between were able to praise the book without first having to debate the appropriateness of two White men writing it. And people were not out to criticize author Alice Walker for penning the introduction to the tome. There were other examples of cross-cultural collaboration, notably bell hooks's first children's book, *Happy to Be Nappy*. Hooks penned a simple ode to nappy hair and chose a White man to be the illustrator. Although hooks says her ideal candidate would have been a Black female, the point was to find the best artist for the job. Chris Raschka, the illustrator, happened to have a way with watercolors and Black hair. However, another children's book, *Nappy Hair*, written by an African-American poet and professor and championed by a White elementary schoolteacher, did not have the same positive results.

Nappy Backlash

Ruth Sherman, twenty-seven, thought that Carolivia Herron's book *Nappy Hair* would be the perfect piece of kiddie literature to inspire her mostly Black and Latino third-graders to read. Knowing that hair could be a sensitive issue in the Black community, the novice teacher shared the book with some of her Black friends to gauge their response. They all loved it and its affirmations about Black hair, evident in lines like "Her hair was an act of God. An act of God that came straight through Africa." With the book's engaging call-and-response format, Sherman knew she had discovered something special. It was a November day in 1998 when Sherman first brought the book to her Bushwick, Brooklyn, classroom for her kids to read, and unknowingly opened a Pandora's box of problems.

More than fifty parents, only one of whom actually had a child in Sherman's classroom, protested and threatened the teacher with physical harm after they saw some photocopied pages of the book that Sherman had distributed to her students. Judging solely on the out-of-context black-and-white copies, the parents deemed *Nappy Hair* racially insulting and culturally insensitive. To make matters worse, since Sherman was a young blond, White woman, many irate parents assumed she was completely unaware of the tumultuous history of Black hair in this country. As the uproar picked up steam and media attention, some of the parents took time out from calling for Sherman's immediate dismissal to read the book. Once they realized that it was not filled with stereotypical caricatures of Buckwheats and pickaninnies and was instead not only harmless but celebratory, they backed off from their blood hunt. Sherman, however, had been through enough at P.S. 75. Worried about her safety, she resigned and asked for reassignment to another school district.

Nappy Hair was based on the author's childhood memory of her uncle telling a story at a family gathering about her "fuzziest, most screwed up, squeezed up, knotted up, tangled up, twisted up, nappy hair." Herron used the tale to explore poetry and the African-American oral tradition of call-and-response. Upon the book's release it sold a mere ten thousand copies. After the Bushwick incident, sales soared to one hundred thousand copies. Media outlets around the world covered the situation because of the shocking display of emotions over a children's book. Yet few outside of the Black community understood the real story.

The *Nappy Hair* uproar was the culmination of generations of Black people's secrecy, frustration, and defensiveness over their hair, coupled with a stance of nationalist protectiveness in all matters concerning it. The Brooklyn parents were not the only ones upset about *Nappy Hair*. Some African-American academicians and literary critics objected to Herron giving racist Whites linguistic ammunition against Blacks through her exploration of the word *nappy*. Other Blacks complained that the word itself was negative, offensive, and hurtful and had no place inside the classroom. Author bell hooks thought that the book would be harmful to any Black child's self-esteem: "There's not one positive comment in the entire book. . . . It's like you're told all these negative things about yourself and by the end you're jumping for joy? Well, that's bullshit and it doesn't happen."

Had the parents of the Bushwick school actually read the book and not just allowed their rage to erupt over the thought of a White woman telling their children about nappiness, would they have perhaps applauded Sherman's efforts at multiculturalism? Had Sherman been fully aware of the almost four hundred years of history behind the word *nappy*, would she have chosen another book and avoided the situation altogether? Whatever outcomes there could have been, the outcry over *Nappy Hair* was a wake-up call for liberals, intellectuals, and laypeople who had come to believe that America had moved significantly toward the celebration of a Black aesthetic, broadening its notions of beauty, and that Blacks had broken free from the anger and shame that surrounded so much of their hair culture.

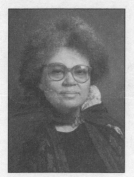

Carolivia Herron,
"The caped, napped
crusader." Courtesy of
Carolivia Herron.

Q&A with the Superhero of Nappy Hair: Carolivia Herron, Author of the Children's Book *Nappy Hair*

Is *nappy* a naughty word?
No, of course not. I know that other people feel it is negative, [but] to me it's such a positive word. It has always been a delight for my family to talk about my hair and how nappy it is. Nappy was definitely a term of endearment.

Just how nappy is your hair?
My hair was so nappy that even though I lived in a 100 percent Black neighborhood [as a child] and most of us had nappy hair, I had to go to another neighborhood on the bus to find a hairdresser who could straighten my kind of hair. Even then it wouldn't straighten. There was a joke in my family: my hair would burn before it would straighten. I like that resistance. No matter what you to do to it, it's going to go back on you.

Was your nappy hair hard to handle?
I don't remember my mother making a big deal about it. It was certainly tedious for her to comb it out. But she was also the one mother in the neighborhood with the lightest hand, and kids even with straight hair would come to her to get it combed because she could take out the tangles without the pain. So I never had any pain associated with it, which many little girls do.

When did you first experience the power of your own nappy hair?
In seventh-grade biology they showed us a picture of the human brain with the little curlicues on the surface. I always thought the little curlicues in my case were so strong they kept going right up to the scalp and kept going up, essentially to God. To me they were going up to God in a beautiful, strong way. The power of creation is the way I would put it.

At the end of the twentieth century, do you think Black people are still ashamed of their naps?
That would be the first thought to come to mind. I had a little boy a couple of weeks ago . . . when I told him I was going to read him the book *Nappy Hair,* he said, "We don't have

nappy hair." And I said, "What do you mean?" And he said, "I was born with it but I don't have it now because they cut it all off so I won't get it." It was like a disease. He looked at me with this innocent face. He had no idea that he still had nappy hair. In a situation like that, what can I do? I just told him, "I love your hair. I love it so much I wish I had some of it."

Would you volunteer to be a nappy hair superhero?
I have no problem with the term, but it's not a name I'd give myself. . . . But when I was in Detroit [at a convention] I had on a *Nappy Hair* T-shirt, my cape behind me, and my African cane. As I was walking through the booths, one woman jumped out of her booth and said, "There goes the caped, napped crusader."

But you've kind of been forced to become the public defender of nappy hair.
Sometimes I feel I've been placed in the role. There are times that I have to remind various people that my prime goal really is art. I'm saying be proud because of the beautiful art we create and I *show* you the great art we create through the celebration of our hair.

How do you feel about your hair today?
I love my hair in its Afro. I don't want it to move. I feel like it resists. It can't be blown around. It's like a halo, like antennae, like some idea that started in the soul and couldn't stop so it had to keep on going until it found its conclusion back in the source of creation. That's what my hair is for me.

Carolivia Herron is a former professor of English at Chico State University in California. Currently Dr. Herron is dedicating herself to developing on-line educational tools and teaching children and adults to appreciate hair, art, and *Star Trek*.

⊙◎⊙◎⊙◎⊙◎⊙◎⊙◎⊙◎⊙◎⊙◎⊙◎⊙◎⊙◎⊙◎⊙◎⊙

"The hair functions as a key ethnic signifier," wrote Kobena Mercer. "Caught on the cusp between self and society, nature and culture, the malleability of hair makes it a sensitive area of expression." And as the *Nappy Hair* fiasco showed the world, Black Americans were still, by 1998, *hypersensitive* about their tresses.

Natural Hair under Attack

The *Nappy Hair* showdown was only the latest in a series of insidious goings-on regarding Black hair. A 1999 *New York Times* article written in response to the situation in Bushwick quoted bell hooks's assertion, "[America] is in the middle of a blond backlash to the multicultural beauty ethos." While hooks was commenting specifically on the rising number of Blacks dying their hair blond, she was also alluding to broader trends toward further dismantling of the lessons of the Black Pride movement. It appeared as though the twentieth century was set to end still upholding the oppressive notions of beauty that had dictated the hair culture of Black America since slavery.

Lauryn Hill, Erykah Badu, and Maxwell may have mainstreamed natural hairstyles in the nineties, but many Blacks and Whites still viewed expressions of kinky hair as problematic and undesirable. Outside the East Coast (especially New York), California, college campuses, and artists' communities, it is still uncommon to find anyone other than children experimenting with natural hairstyles. By 1997, according to an AHBAI survey, one in four Black women had some form of hair add-on, with the figure expected to rise to one in three. African-Americans spend $225 million annually on hair-weaving services and products. Approximately two-thirds of all Black women wore their hair straightened, by either hot combs or chemical relaxers. There was a resurgence of Black men getting their hair texturized (a mild relaxer) or straightened—including high-profile celebrities like comedian Chris Rock and music mogul Sean "Puffy" Combs (who appeared in a cover story in a 1999 *GQ* magazine with hair styled similarly to the slick, conked *Quo Vadis* cut of the late 1950s). So many Americans still use some sort of process to alter their hair texture that hair expert Willie Morrow predicts that one day the Black race will be bald from all the chemicals.

This continued popularity of long, straight, and generally un-nappy hair could simply be read as aesthetic preference, yet both within and outside of the Black community, natural hairstyles are still under attack. Natural, unstraightened looks that display Black hair textures are generally perceived as "too ethnic," "too Black," or an aggressive challenge to middle-class American values. Often the harshest critics are other Black people.

Many parents and older generation Blacks maintain that unstraight hair will infringe on their children's and grandchildren's chances for economic and social survival. The same young men who sparked the resurgence in cornrows and Afros—often in emulation of their favorite athletes—were unable to find after-school employment because of their "thuggish" appearance. While corporate America accepts yarmulkes, turbans, and other ethnic or religious signifiers, dredlocs and other Black hairstyles are often seen as signs of militance and anger. Black men working in these environments typically find it necessary to keep their haircuts conservative and short, making sure that no naps are able to peek through. Nelson Boyce, the happily dredloced advertising director, appears to be the exception, not the rule. Dredlocs, nearly two decades after being introduced to the United States, still evoke images in many Black and White Americans of drug users, drug dealers, dirtiness, and militancy.

During the late nineties, even small children were being called to task for some of their hairstyles. In 1996, third-grader Megan Smith was sent home from Grace Christian School in Saint Petersburg, Florida, and told not to return until she changed her "extreme" hairstyle. Her multibraided style was said to clash "with the spiritual and educational mission" of the private school because—along with other "extreme" styles like dredlocs, dyed hair, and "gaudy" hair ornaments—it was seen as a distraction to other students. One month earlier at a suburban Chicago school, Rickover Junior High, administrators pulled twelve-year-old TaCara Nash and thirteen-year-old Aqueelah Shareef out of class and gave the two girls a choice of all-day isolated detention or going home. Both students had arrived at school that day with a zigzag part in their hair. Apparently the zigzag part fell into the category of "carved symbols in the head," which were banned under the school district's antigang policy. Other hairstyles linked with "gang looks" included cornrows, dredlocs, and ponytails (on boys). In a school district that was 54 percent White, 34 percent Black, and 11 percent Latino, a multiracial contingent of parents protested that the overwhelming number of banned styles were "Black." The policy was eventually updated, and cornrows, dredlocs, and braids were allowed, although haircuts and head carvings displaying patterns, signs, symbols, or words were still prohibited.

Predominantly White schools were not the only organizations policing the appropriateness of Black natural hairstyles. In 1998 seventeen-year-old North Carolinian Michelle Barksile had been invited to be a debutante in a Black sorority ball. But Barksile wore her hair in shoulder-length dredlocs, and the Alpha Kappa Alpha sorority advised the debutante-to-be that she would need to pin up her hair on the night of the ball. Barksile, who likened her hair to rays of sun, refused to comply, because she thought the prescribed style would make her look like animated TV mom Marge Simpson. When Barksile said that she would not adjust her hair, the invitation was revoked and her hopes of following in her mother's footsteps as a debutante were dashed.

The story made national and international headlines. Only weeks after the *Nappy Hair* incident, Black America's hair issues were once again being exposed and dissected before the world. Barksile appeared on the national talk show *Leeza* and turned down numerous invitations from other programs. She said the experience had taught her never to alter herself to fit others' standards. One AKA sorority sister, Ruby P. Greene, wrote to the Raleigh *News & Observer* to give her opinion on what she saw as Barksile's "regrettable" decision. Greene maintained that the sorority did not condemn natural hairstyles but insisted that they be "neat, clean, well groomed and . . . quite elegant." She also wrote that "dredlocs are not culturally significant to the Black [American] experience." Apparently Greene saw a pinned-up French roll as more culturally Black. Many Americans of all races disagreed with Greene's reasoning and saw the sorority's actions as both regressive and elitist.

American Beauty

While natural hair was not universally desired at the end of millennium, many Black Americans were still searching for a way to "improve" their hair naturally. In a clear case of history repeating itself, a product was introduced to the market in 1999 that promised a *natural*, chemical-free way to get "hair that moves." Using the same marketing scheme as Rio, the disaster product of the early nineties, this new miracle cure was called Copa. Via a late-night infomercial featuring product endorser and entertainer Debbie Allen and her dredloced hairstylist Snacky, the 96 percent natural Copa "curl release system" promised to "give you freedom. Freedom from the effects of humidity, freedom to work out or swim."

Perhaps still recalling the photos of Rio victims' patchy bald heads and sandwich bags full of hair, Black women have not embraced Copa in great numbers. But the very existence of the product underlines the rut that Black America stays in regarding hair. "Freedom" is still equated with having straight hair. Neither the product's infomercial nor the other hair straightening systems on the market mention that women and men with braids, dredlocs, and various natural styles have the freedom to swim, sweat, and walk in the rain without destroying their styles. The reason for the omission is that these manufacturers understand that the majority of Blacks would not see freedom in wearing natural hair. They would instead feel further alienated, ostracized, and unattractive.

Black men's and women's psyches still value unkinky hair much more than the type that grows out of most Black heads. Popular culture continues to be filled with Black women with long, or at least soft, moving hair. Music videos overflow with light-skinned, long-haired women or, continuing a trend that started in the early nineties, feature women who are of mixed heritage, Asian or Latina. Beauty advertising historically preys on the insecurities of those in its intended market, and the Black hair game is no exception. Since the days of the first Black newspapers, advertisements have told Black people that their hair is unacceptable and downright ugly. In 1998 a billboard campaign was introduced for Bone Strait Relaxer system. The ad showed a woman with long, straight hair, her head slightly arched back. The caption read, "My Hair. Your Man. His Fingers. Your Drama." It became a source of outrage for many (of all races) who felt that the campaign lacked cutural sensitivity and portrayed Black women as sexually licentious home-wreckers. African-Americans expressed their disapproval of the campaign that so insidiously linked having long, straight, touchable hair with having not only a man but someone else's man. In a culture where women were continually made to feel that they were attractive primarily if they fit into a certain beauty mold, this ad hit a raw nerve with those Black women who always worried that no man would find their hair "touchable" and beautiful.

Ironically, the campaign was created and executed by Spike/BBDO, the ad company co-owned by filmmaker Spike Lee—the same man who once forced Black Americans to face their color and hair issues in his film *School Daze*. A spokesperson for the agency said that the ad was meant as "fun" and to show the "playful gamesmanship that exists between Black women." But surely the company knew that Black women find few things funny about hair, and even less when it comes to their men. Company spokesperson Charles Hall further explained that while the ad may have been low-brow "Jerry Springer" type humor, it was not meant as a statement on how to take someone's man.

Children, who pick up their cultural cues from family and schoolmates, still favor long, straight hair. As bell hooks notes, "Every day of our lives in this society a Black child somewhere is slaughtering their hair with dangerous products." In recent years, little Black girls have been wearing their hair in braid extensions that often fall past the middle of their backs. Parents typically claim that the style shaves tremendous time off the morning routine. But many social critics and commentators see danger in adding long, un-kinky hair to the heads of little girls who must develop an ethnic identity and self-esteem in a society that looks down on short, nappy tresses. It is seen as a way of telling these children from a very early age that what they naturally possess must somehow be amended in order to be pretty and acceptable.

America's, including Black America's, beauty ideal has not altered drastically since the late 1800s. Large breasts, small waists, and masses of flowing hair are still the look desired by men and sought after by many women. The adoption of certain Black looks and trends by Whites does not indicate a more inclusive definition of beauty but merely offers Whites a broader range of ways to look "exotic" or "different." Black people looking to fit into the mainstream visually still overwhelmingly have to contend with the same standards as in the past.

More than one hundred years after the terms "good" and "bad" hair became part of the Black American lexicon, the concepts endure. Those who grew up during the Black Pride movement of the sixties and seventies have children who must now contend with the same problems. Teens today use the concepts of "good" and "bad" hair, learning about them from their friends, family, schoolmates, and the media. While many teens think that some natural styles are attractive on certain people ("You have to have the face for it," warns one Pennsylvania sixteen-year-old), straight hair is the norm. "Good hair is the type of hair that doesn't get out of control even if you haven't had a perm in months," explains Rhode Island teen Toni Ashford, fifteen. "It's when you can go swimming and keep on steppin' and still look a'ight. I learned about this concept when I was five when I realized that I didn't have good hair . . . the day of my first perm."

Toward the Future . . .

Some time after the Brooklyn school debacle, a Dallas librarian, Guinea Bennett (who wears her own hair unstraightened and in a puffy ponytail), read *Nappy Hair* to a group of kindergartners at a public library story hour. Before she opened the pages of the book, Bennett asked the children to define *nappy hair*, and one young Black boy answered, "When your hair is messed up." When Bennett pointed out that her own hair was nappy and then asked the children what they thought of it, the kids responded that it was pretty. The librarian then inquired, "Can nappy hair be pretty?" The resounding reply was an excited "Yes!" The group then settled down and listened attentively as Bennett read them the tale of little Brenda and her nappy locs.

Ten Memorable Moments in Black Hair History

Circa 1845: The hot comb is invented in France.

1910: The first year hair-care entrepreneur Madam C. J. Walker makes the *Guinness Book of World Records* as the first Black self-made female millionaire.

1948: Mexican chemist Jose Calva discovers that the same process that turns sheep's wool into mink-like fur can turn kinky hair straight.

1969: The year Angela Davis's image—massive Afro on display—is disseminated to the masses by the FBI. Warning: Afroed and dangerous.

1981: The proud lady symbol, reminding consumers to buy Black, is introduced by the American Health and Beauty Aids Institute.

January 27, 1984: Michael Jackson's hair catches fire during the shooting of a Pepsi commercial.

July 1989: Quaker Oats removes Aunt Jemima's signature red headrag and updates her look with a no-lye relaxer.

November 1998: The first Madam C. J. Walker commemorative stamp is issued by the U.S. Postal Service.

Later in November 1998: A White teacher in Brooklyn is threatened with bodily harm for reading the book *Nappy Hair* to her third-grade students. She eventually leaves the school, fearing for her safety. The book goes on to sell a hundred thousand copies.

January 26, 1999: Tennis star Venus Williams receives a point penalty and subsequently loses at the Australian Open semi-finals when some of her trademark beads fly off her braids and onto the court.

8

The Divided Decade:
The Early 2000s

In the early years of the twenty-first century, the Internet proved itself to be the greatest contribution to Black hair culture since the hot comb. "It was a total game changer," says Michaela Angela Davis, an image activist who works to expand the narrow lens of how Black women are depicted. Davis is right. Never before had Black people, and women in particular, had the means to be in such direct, informative, daily conversation with each other about this loaded topic. And while the Internet had indeed changed daily life globally—revolutionizing the way that people shop, get news, and communicate with each other—its effects on Black hair have been more far-reaching than anyone could have imagined.

Eighty-one percent of American adults were on the Internet regularly, including 23.9 million African-Americans. A substantial 70 percent of Black women were online, with a sizable number watching instructional videos on

YouTube, buying hair products, reading blogs with product reviews, and posting photos on Instagram of other women with amazing hair. In sum, Black women had incorporated the Internet into their arsenal of beauty tools. "Through YouTube and social media, Black women are in conversation with each other. It has given us education, power and agency," says Davis. Now in the same way that women of all races would talk publicly about their weight, Black people were having public conversations about their hair.

Yet these conversations have also provided a platform that showed the lingering hold of some of the culture's most troubling hair demons. Simply because America was in the early days of a new century did not mean that it had freed itself from traumas of the past. And so through these online interactions and the rising number of public discussions in other media outlets, what distinguishes the first years of the new millennium is that it was a time of extreme difference in philosophies in Black hair culture: an era of great pride in natural hair textures, an explosion in the number of women wearing weaves (and claiming it with no hint of shame or secrecy), and bitter, angry Hair Policing over what was considered "respectable" and "appropriate." It is easy to see why the beginning of the twenty-first century will be remembered as the divided decade, a time of contrasting views and philosophies on what was right and wrong about Black hair.

#teamnatural Takes Over

In the very first years of the twenty-first century, Black women quietly started embracing their natural hair texture, rejecting the relaxers they'd been wearing for years. But before Black women went natural, the whole country went green.

It may have started when recycling went from being a radical concept to a legal requirement in neighborhoods across America. Or it may have been the increased media coverage on water scarcity, pollution, and the destruction of the ozone layer, followed by Al Gore's sobering 2006 documentary on climate change, *An Inconvenient Truth*. People wanted to alter the course of Mother Nature's impending path toward destruction. They were eager to change their ways, and the "change" people grabbed hold of was "going green" or "living naturally." By the middle of the first decade of the twenty-first century, the American public was hooked on this new natural lifestyle. What's more, the derogatory 1990s image of a wild-eyed, antiestablishment tree hugger as the symbol of an environmental activist had been replaced by a stay-at-home mom turned organic baby-food purveyor.

Product manufacturers tried to stay ahead of the movement by offering everything from toilet paper to laundry detergent in a "greener" version so people could be eco-conscious without having to give up their favorite consumer products. Soon enough, everybody was doing it. And it—from shopping with canvas grocery bags to composting last night's leftovers—became less of a sacrifice and more of a new trend. And hair care was right in the mix.

For many Black women, going green initially meant buying shampoos and conditioners that didn't contain harmful ingredients like sodium lauryl sulfate and parabens. But soon her lifestyle was also being overhauled beyond shopping choices. Yoga, herbal teas, and a diet that no longer included fast food or red meat became common. So, of course it came to pass that these same women began to question their hair-care practices, particularly those who straightened their hair with chemical relaxers. "I felt this overwhelming urge to come clean and get back to myself," says Texas native Jesaline Berry about her decision to go natural. "I was coming to terms with the fact that I had been subjecting myself to all of those toxic chemicals for all of those years."

Though these women may have felt like the only one in their town, office, or social organization without a relaxer in the early 2000s, they were actually part a growing, though still not widely visible, trend. Alongside these women—drops of natural hair in a bucket of relaxers, weaves, and wigs—there were cultural thinkers like journalist Lisa Jones and braider/documentarian Yvette Smalls, who were writing books, making movies, and leading workshops to discuss the power and meaning of Black hair. And the public was in love with singers like India.Arie, Jill Scott, and Erykah Badu, whose natural hairstyles offered alternatives to the Black celebrity beauty standard.

There was also Alicia Keys, who in 2001 became a music superstar with the release of her debut album *Songs in A Minor*. She did photo shoots and toured the world with an always-changing cornrowed hairstyle, each more intricate than the last. "Alicia was aligning herself—in style and substance—with her musical foremothers including Patrice Rushen and Nina Simone, both of whom rocked beautiful, soulful cornrows," says

Karen Good Marable, a journalist who has written about the history of cornrows. "She wasn't just using hair as trend and art form, but also branding and identity."

Even on television, women found a natural hair icon to admire. Tracee Ellis Ross is Diana's daughter, an unapologetic fashion diva and natural hair–wearer who starred on the popular prime-time sitcom *Girlfriends*, which ran from 2000 to 2008. Ross played Joan Clayton, a meticulous, type-A personality and attorney-turned-restaurateur. As uptight as Joan was, her hair—a mass of curls and spirals—was the complete opposite. It was the first time, since braided lawyer Maxine on *Living Single*, that natural hair had gone so corporate. Ross's hair defied typical casting decisions and helped to expand people's ideas about who wore natural hair. During the eight years the show aired, Ross's voluminous, bouncy curls soon became as adored as the series.

In addition to this handful of natural-haired celebrities, there was a new magazine on the scene that was committed to showing and celebrating Black beauty differently than the other women's publications on the market. *Honey*, launched in 1999, had a dredloced Lauryn Hill on the cover of its preview issue and in the following years consistently featured natural hair alongside straight styles and weaves. Norell Giancana, Ph.D., a sociologist who examined *Honey* for her doctoral dissertation on how Black women represent themselves, says, "Like the very early days of *Essence*, *Honey* showed Black women in a variety of ways. There was no judgment about straight or natural hair."

Honey's founding editors, Joicelyn Dingle and Kierna Mayo, did this intentionally after years of disappointment in how other publications covered Black hair. "Magazines are sacrosanct to me," says Dingle. "Before *Honey*, one of my favorites was [the now-defunct] *Mademoiselle*. One month, they did a story on the history of braids. They managed to print the story without one photo of a Black model. I sent a long letter to the editor. How can you talk about the history of braids and not mention Africa? Soon after they did a story on dredlocs. The opening page was a photo of a Puli, the dog with corded hair, followed by four White women with locs and a Black model who didn't have locs but very short twists. I was on fire. Instead of writing another letter, I wrote a business plan."

Picking up on these cultural cues around them, young Black women started reconsidering their ideas of beauty when it came to their hair. Going natural, like Alicia Keys or Tracee Ellis Ross, didn't seem radical. Natural hair was no longer as foreign to the notion of what was beautiful. "Women didn't have to feel like an outlier if they went natural," says editor-in-chief of *Essence* magazine Vanessa Bush.

And the Internet was there to help them with their new look. In the past, if a woman stopped using a relaxer, she was left with many questions about how to care for her natural hair. Often her friends, family, and even former hairstylist would look at her cluelessly, as

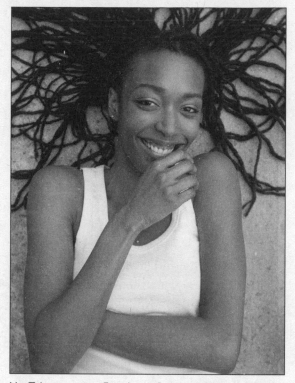

YouTube sensation Franchesca Ramsey. (Photo credit: Leslie Harrler Studio)

they only knew about relaxed hair. So she would be forced to become a stealth detective, stopping women on the street who had natural hair and peppering them with endless questions. And she would pour hundreds of dollars into products that she prayed would work but which often ended up unused.

That's what happened to Franchesca Ramsey, a graphic designer and social media/marketing consultant. In 2004 she did the Big Chop, the new millennium phrase for cutting off all of her relaxed hair. Then her mother's friend helped her begin growing locs. Soon after, she was off to her freshman year of college with the meager budget of a student who could not afford regular salon visits. "I didn't know what to do," says Ramsey. Fortunately chat rooms were the newest phenomenon to hit the Internet. These virtual spaces let members gather to discuss everything from dating to video games to, Ramsey was pleased to learn, hair. "I joined a forum called

Get Up, Dread Up," she explains, adding that she was one of just three Black people on the site. "It was all White people talking about their dreds and how to care for them. So a lot of the advice—like using beeswax—didn't work for me, but I stayed a member of the group."

Ramsey was inspired by Get Up, Dread Up. It became clear to her that people wanted a space where they could learn about their locs and how to care for them. So in 2007 she started posting pictures of her hair online, soon moving on to video tutorials about how to style and care for her locs. "I didn't see anyone else doing it, so I did," she explains pragmatically.

And though Ramsey does not consider herself a hair expert, tens of thousands flock online to Chescalocs, her YouTube channel where she posts videos about her hair. Some of the topics are basic how-tos, while others show off Ramsey's sense of humor, including "The Secret to Long Natural Hair" (her tongue-in-cheek answer: patience).

By 2013, there were thousands of blogs about Black hair. Twitter, Facebook, and YouTube also had countless pages and channels dedicated to discussing its significance, care, and versatility. On these sites were articles; photos; videos and podcasts about products; step-to-step how-tos on creating styles; and essays, opinion boards, and think pieces on issues that natural hair women have grappled with on the job and in their personal lives.

Gone were the days of feeling alone if you didn't have a relaxer, thanks in large part to the communities formed by these thousands of women who created, read, and supported natural hair sites online. "I had been a creamy crack addict most of my life and needed to reeducate myself on products, techniques, and styles," says Cynthia Winder, a fifty-five-year-old woman from Baltimore who began to visit natural hair sites after she gave up the "creamy crack," or hair relaxer. "These sites kept me inspired and encouraged that I could do this natural hair thing."

Through this online community, a culture developed. It went by the Twitter handle #teamnatural and had its own vocabulary to describe styles and grooming techniques. Harnessing the power of the Internet, #teamnatural also brought women together offline in a variety of often creative ways. There were meetups, which are gatherings held at homes, salons, or lounges, where anywhere from a dozen to hundreds of "naturalistas" could have face-to-face conversations with each other. There were also panels organized around topics like "What Men Think About Natural Hair" and

"Natural Hair Goes to Work." In addition, women could go to natural hair shows, Happy to Be Nappy parties and demonstrations on styles. There were even natural hair cruises, like the Showing My Roots Cruise, where women could travel to island locales and keep talking about their hair. Essentially, any idea that was centered around natural hair was guaranteed a healthy attendance of interested women, proving the organizing power and wide reach of #teamnatural.

Natural hair had moved into the beauty conversation in ways it never had before. After twenty-six years spent doing hair, stylist and author of *Textured Tresses: The Ultimate Guide to Maintaining and Styling Natural Hair* Diane Da Costa says, "Natural hair was now about expression and creativity. It wasn't a political statement but more of a trend and about fashion." Vanessa Bush from *Essence* agrees. "I think the whole natural revolution is a reflection of where we are in our own self-acceptance in a way. It's about being comfortable in your own skin. And it really makes me smile to know that a new generation of Black women get to experience that freedom."

Black Hair According to Chris Rock

Chris Rock has gained millions of fans and made millions of dollars by making people laugh. Yet he couldn't find anything humorous about the moment when his young daughter came to him in tears, asking why she did not have "good hair." This is a question that many parents have been asked behind closed doors for generations in Black families, but Rock decided to answer it publicly—and with major corporate backing. He secured cable channel giant HBO to come on board as a producer. Then he embarked upon a journey to understand why his daughter was so distraught, and traveled to eight locations, interviewing dozens of people. What he learned became the 2009 documentary *Good Hair*.

"Secrets will rot the soul, they're good for no one," Rock told *USA Today* for an article about the film's theatrical release. So he gathered celebrities, some of the planet's most secretive people when it comes to beauty routines, to get honest while the cameras rolled. Actress Nia Long admitted that she has a pool but doesn't swim in it because of her hair; there was also self-described "weave connoisseur" and former child star Raven-Symoné, rappers Salt-N-Pepa, natural-haired actress Tracie Thorns, poet laureate Maya Angelou, and others who offered their insights into why Black women spend so much time and money on their hair. The crew visited the Bronner Bros. hair show in Atlanta and a temple in India that provides a substantial amount of the hair imported into the U.S. to turn into weaves. Rock, of course, got to be the Funny Man, cracking jokes at a barbershop and various other places on this Black Hair Tour.

Suddenly, because of *Good Hair*, words like "creamy crack" were being used in the pages of *USA Today; The New York Times* was holding roundtable discussions on Black women and hair and publishing articles that pondered "why some African-American women feel they need long, silky, straight hair to fit into White society." White America may have been left wide-eyed by some of the information given in the film, which went on to win a Special Jury Prize at Sundance and gross $4,157,104 dollars—yet many Black women were giving Rock and his all-male group of producers and writers the side eye.

Teresa Wiltz, columnist for Black-interest Web site The Root, wrote, "There are two things that [Rock] does not bring to the conversation: Context and compassion." In its place there was a scant one mention—positioned an hour into a 96-minute film—of the phrase "self-esteem" and no thorough examination of beauty politics or White supremacy or the lingering effects of slavery in America.

Entertainment Weekly columnist Alynda Wheat wrote that the film, "doesn't offer a cogent, relevant analysis of why Black women relax their hair or wear extensions—which was supposed to have been the point." Instead, some argued, it showed Black women as financially reckless, spending rent money on their hair. It was, apparently, a problem of such magnitude that civil rights activist Reverend Al Sharpton took to public admonishment, telling the cameras, "How do you have a thousand-dollar weave on but don't have money in your house to feed your kids?" The documentary also trotted out the gold-digger stereotype that has plagued Black women throughout American history, in multiple scenes where men claim they pay for their girlfriend's or wife's weave even though it is hard on their working-class pockets. "The price of maintaining a woman is like real estate in New York . . . it's skyrocketing!" said media mogul Andre Harrell about the costs of weaves and the hair salon. Other viewers and critics were upset that a scene that shows that the chemical found in relaxer cream is so potent it can disintegrate a soda can was immediately followed by a scene of a six-year-old girl getting that very same cream applied to her young scalp.

Yet even with the detractors, Chris Rock struck gold with *Good Hair*. The box office numbers pleased HBO, and countless Black people were also happy to see a part of their culture get the Hollywood treatment. It gave a financial boost to the stylists, barbers, and other hair-care professionals who were featured in the film.

Furthermore, many agreed with Rock that there was no way to move past the painful side of hair culture if people did not talk, talk, and talk some more. "This was a conversation normally happening behind closed doors," says comedian W. Kamau Bell, who credits *Good Hair* with being a step in the right direction regarding Black hair culture in the new millennium. "The more of those conversations Black people can have with each other, the better." In addition, the film drew White people into the conversation. "After *Good Hair* came out, a lot more White people—including ones I'd known for a long time—suddenly felt comfortable talking to me about my hair," says Jennifer Michaels, forty, a mother of three who wears her shoulder-length hair in dredlocs. "Unfortunately, they all assumed I was wearing a weave, even though my hair doesn't look like something you'd pay for."

Weaves Gone Wild

While chemical relaxers get their share of abuse in *Good Hair*, Rock spends much of the film skewering weaves. "They always say diamonds are a girl's best friend, but diamonds better watch out because there's a new friend in town and its name is weave," Rock says in the movie, adding later that women are "more hooked on [weaves] than, say, cocaine." *Good Hair* was on to something: By 2009, the year of its release, weaves were everywhere. They were on TV, in movies, at the post office, the supermarket. They were, in fact, nearly any place where you could find a Black woman. (Though to be fair, White women were also loving the weave.) Even women who wanted natural styles were getting in on the trend, simultaneously blurring the line of what it meant to be "natural" while increasing the profits of the weave industry. And these women who embraced the weave were doing it without the shame or secrecy that was typical just ten years earlier, when one of the greatest insults was to ask someone, "Is that *your* hair?"

"In the beginning, weaves were not something you talked about," says Mimi Valdés, former editor-in-chief of *Vibe Vixen* magazine, which ran an article on the history of the hair weave in its 2004 debut issue as a nod to the growing trend. "They were considered a bad thing. Yet by the early 2000s, they were commonplace, the default hairstyle—especially for celebrities." This new generation of weave lovers included almost every Black female star of the time, including models Tyra Banks and Selita Ebanks, singers like Beyoncé, Mary J. Blige, and Mariah Carey, actresses Gabrielle Union, Angela Bassett, Sanaa Lathan, and the list goes on and on and on. Adrin Seven Washington, who specializes in hair extensions at his Bethesda, Maryland, salon Seven and Company, explains, "No one wanted fake hair. But the more people wore them it was, 'Oh, a celeb has it on, I can wear one.'" Washington, who has worked with singer Chaka Khan, explains that the reason women want weaves is simple: freedom! "You don't have to do your hair every day, you wake up and the weave already looks good," he says.

For Tammy Chichester, a thirty-two-year-old Temple Hill, Maryland, office manager for a doctor's office, there is no shame at all in her weave game. "I change my weave once every three to four weeks," she says, noting that she mainly wears them for styling ease, but also likes them for fun. "Right now I have a curly style for the season. I mostly get inspired by the weather, and this summer I want to go curly so it won't be a big deal to get it wet in the pool. But I also wear short bobs, curly and long, side parts, parts down the middle, full weaves, partial weaves, cap weaves, blond, black, red, brown, everything!" It would be impossible for any one person to naturally have such a revolving door of styles, so Chichester doesn't even try to pretend.

By the middle of the decade, weaves

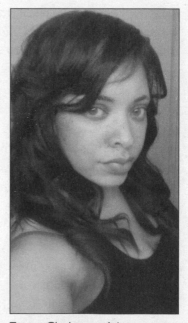

Tammy Chichester of the ever-changing weaves. (Courtesy of subject)

had become so popular that one famous Black woman was ready to jump into the conversation with both feet and zero weave tracks. Supermodel-turned-TV-mogul Tyra Banks was on a mission to debunk the idea that weaves were necessary in order to be considered beautiful, so she declared September 8, 2009, National Real Hair Day.

This holiday did not involve a parade or vacation time from work, but it did get an entire hour of attention on national television. A press release Tyra issued in advance of the show read, "We're taking it to the next level and getting more real than ever before by encouraging women everywhere to own and rock what they've got and be proud! For the Season 5 premiere, I will be doing just that—no fake hair, I'm rocking my REAL hair. . . . We welcome everyone to go natural with me!"

So September 8 arrived and the first glimpse of Tyra on the show was of the former model emerging out of the shower, albeit in full makeup, with her chemically straightened hair wet and unstyled. She walked confidently onto the stage in a jumpsuit, stilettos, and the same wet hair, turning around so the audience could see that it came only to her shoulders and did not hang down her back. For the next hour, Tyra and other guests showed how good they looked without extensions and why everyone could feel just as beautiful without add-ons.

Some, however, felt they had been bamboozled by Real Hair Day. Blogger Patrice Yursik of the popular beauty Web site Afrobella confessed on her blog that she had wrongly taken "real" to mean "natural" when what Tyra meant was simply "no weave." She wrote, "Tyra's 'Real Hair Day' was the beginning of an important conversation. But myself and the many natural-haired women I know were left cold by the episode. Where were the women with kinky, coily, natural hair textures?"

Yursik wasn't the only one left disappointed, yet Tyra's episode highlighted a new conflict in Black hair culture. Because of the widespread trend of weaves and hairpieces, fake hair was the new norm—so by not wearing it, could one arguably be called "natural"? Though her "Real Hair Day" did garner high ratings for Banks, it also highlighted a growing rift between #teamnatural and others, whether it was women with straight styles or, more often, people who expressed negative opinions about natural hair.

#teamnatural Takes on the World

"In the nineties, natural women felt 'if you have a weave, you are not a real sister,'" says image activist Davis, who has been natural since the 1990s. "But this new generation is freer." They were also vigilant, using the Internet—and the #teamnatural hashtag on Twitter—to virally shame people or institutions that said negative things about natural hair. For example, when Shreveport, Louisiana, meteorologist Rhonda Lee was fired in 2013 for responding to a viewer's comment that she should switch her short Afro to a straight style, the news did not get much press—until #teamnatural caught wind of it. Bloggers and their readers kept the story alive by not just reporting on what happened but also by calling for petitions and protests against the station that did not grant Lee free speech to defend her natural hair.

#teamnatural also came to the defense of celebrities when necessary. When singer Solange Knowles went natural, replacing the weave that fans had long grown accustomed to seeing her wear, many outside the natural hair community made critical comments. Beyoncé's younger sister, Knowles, cut her hair in July 2009 and became the number-three trending topic on Twitter, placing her ahead of the presidential elections in Iran and President Obama's new healthcare plan. Solange was accused of being "insane" and "doing a Britney," recalling the time when pop star Spears shaved off her hair during a period of extreme mental stress. Few of the critics seemed to care that Solange had been spending what she estimated to be $40,000–$50,000 per year on weaves. Nor did it seem to register when she said on *Oprah* that she didn't feel as pretty without a weave, and that pre-cut she was in hair "bondage." To the naysayers, this amount of money and those negative feelings didn't matter—what mattered was that she no longer had straight, long hair. Meanwhile, her most vocal defenders, from #teamnatural, elevated Solange to the level of style icon, publicizing and popularizing the short, natural braids, twists, and even natural-textured wigs she would wear. While this celebration of natural styles is a positive move, some, like Atlanta-based celebrity hairstylist Derek J, feel that #teamnatural gets overzealous in their watchdog efforts and have nicknamed them "Natural Nazis."

Another group that the Natural Hair movement monitored frequently through online articles, polls, and YouTube testimonials were Black men because, historically, they have been vocal in not loving natural hair. When Joan Morgan, author of *When Chickenheads Come Home to Roost: A Hip-Hop Feminist Breaks It Down,* was a guest on MSNBC's *Melissa Harris-Perry* show, she said, "Black women's bodies are always in conversation . . . with society and with Black men. It's not just how we think about our hair, it's how we think Black men are going to think about our hair. . . . Are we going to be desirable lovers?"

It is a significant question that has plagued many women when they thought about saying good-bye to straight hair. Writer and relationship expert Demetria L. Lucas wrote a story for The Root titled "Why Does My Natural Hair Get No Love?," where she admitted there was "a healthy chunk of Black guys who prefer . . . for a Black woman's hair to be straight." However, Lucas took the time to put the question of texture to fifty Black men she dubbed her "Male Mind Squad" and wrote that "they all agreed that a woman rocking natural hair is . . . not remotely intimidating, at least not to a man who appreciates a confident woman." Jozen Cummings, the dating editor for the *New York Post*, agrees. Cummings, who is also the creator of Until I Get Married, a personal blog about his dating life as a Black man in his thirties, says that men are not as driven in their quest to date a woman with a certain *texture* of hair, but he admits that one trait still reigns supreme: length. "Long hair is associated with femininity, and a lot of men feel it is a part of their idea of what a woman should look like," says Cummings.

A Good-bye to Good Hair?

Arguably, an added and unintended side effect of the two biggest trends to hit Black hair in the new millennium—weaves and a rise in naturals—was that fewer women were worrying about "good" or "bad" hair. For instance, with weaves so commonplace, instead of a lifetime spent unhappy with her hair texture or length, a woman could stash away some cash and buy any texture or length she desired. With the hair of her dreams just a purchase away, why should "good hair" really matter anymore?

The reality is that it will take more than a few tracks of hair to dismantle over two centuries of entrenched, harmful thinking. "You're still going to have a 'good hair' conversation in certain parts of the country or amongst youth," says Yaba Blay, who is the codirector of the Africana Studies program at Drexel University and author of *(1)ne Drop: Shifting the Lens on Race*, which explores the interconnected nuances of skin color politics and Black racial identity. "Now, though, it may not be good versus bad, but an acknowledgment of—and keening over—'good.'"

Blay's point was exemplified on another 2009 episode of *The Tyra Banks Show*. One season before her Real Hair Day, Banks dedicated an hour-long episode to talking about "good hair." It featured a woman who intentionally married a White man so her children would have "biracial" hair, as well as a mother who chemically straightened her three-year-old's hair. However, for many viewers, the most sobering moment on the show was when a little Black girl explained she always wanted to wear her Hannah Montana wig because the long, blond tresses were prettier, in her mind, than her own hair.

Children, however, were not the only ones still under the influence of "good hair" thinking. And NaKesha Smith became an online hit for pointing out that a good/bad hair mentality exists in one of the most unexpected arenas: the natural hair movement. In 2010, Smith released a video on her popular YouTube channel called "You Natural Hair Girls Make Me Sick!" which claims that there are not enough women with "real African, textured hair" present on the many natural hair sites.

Smith later uploaded a video called "I'm not apologizing for being a 4g." It refers to the designation of hair texture which many #teamnatural blogs and video tutorials used. Back in 1998, Oprah's hairstylist, Andre Walker, wrote the book *Andre Talks Hair*, in which he designated four types of hair based on texture. Working from his designations, the Web site Naturallycurly.com went deeper and set up classifications for varying degrees of non-straight hair—from barely waved to seriously coiled. The numerical system goes from one through four with A, B, and C variations. The straighter the hair, the lower the letter and number. Most Black women fall somewhere between 3B and 4C, though there are many, like Smith, who argue that a substantial amount of natural hair sites spent a lot of time focused on the threes.

These designations can be helpful in a number of ways. For instance, on the popular Web site Black Girl with Long Hair there is an extensive database where readers can search for women by their curl pattern, seeing the styles, products, and other habits that are suited to a texture similar to their own. From a practical standpoint, this is a great way to see what would work and how to best achieve it. Still, placing hair in categories is controversial.

"This vocabulary, the 4A and 4B thing, is interesting and problematic," says Blay. "It is no different than talking about 'grades' of hair. When we talk about the politics of beauty, it is aligned with and reflective of White power and White supremacy. And this exists in the natural hair community."

Valuing certain natural hair over another went hand in hand with dreaming that there was a product that would create what Imani Dawson, creator of natural hair Web site A Tribe Called Curl, calls "big, biracial hair," the often unspoken goal of many who were natural. That with just the right cream or gel they would suddenly look like new millennium hair icon Tracee Ellis Ross. What was rarely discussed was that Ross has a White father, meaning that part of the secret behind her big, bouncy curls was not what she found in a bottle but what was in her gene pool. Some went so far as to use products that were *supposedly* natural to alter their curl or kink pattern but actually included chemicals and could cause damage, such as the Brazilian keratin treatment (which contains formaldehyde).

Not only were there products for elongating a natural hair wearer's curls, there were also "stretching" techniques intended to change the hair's texture. These included flat twists, braid outs, Nubian knots and other textured "sets." "What type of natural hair are we talking about?" asks Blay. "Is it what grows out of your head or a manipulated natural?"

This idea of "manipulated naturals" led to a 2012 *New York Times* story, "How Natural Is Too Natural?" Writer Jessica Andrews quotes Afrobella's Patrice Yursik as saying, "The belief that straighter textures and longer lengths of hair are somehow more beautiful comes from what we see around us. Look at the images of black women in the media—if their hair isn't straight, it's a very particular type of curly look that's meant to represent natural hair. It's another way for the arbiters of mainstream beauty to divide our community."

Divisiveness and hostility over the texture of natural hair was something that Solange Knowles experienced firsthand. After someone sent her a link to an online article about how her hair looked "dry," "unkempt," and even "homeless," she decided she was done being a hair icon to #team-natural. She wrote on Twitter, "I never painted myself as a #teamnatural vice president. I don't know the lingo and I don't sleep with a damn satin cap." And instead of taking the unsolicited styling advice, she let everyone know that she "hates" twist outs and, more to the point, was not talking "about no damn hair . . . no mo."

Even men weren't immune to the valuation of what constituted "good" natural hair. In 2013, when Prince, no stranger to chemically straightened hair, wore his hair in a mini Afro during a performance on the *Billboard* Music Awards, people using the hashtag #teamnatural on Twitter said that what the living legend needed was a twist out to give his 'fro some definition. Unlike Solange, Prince did not respond on social media. Instead, he just ignored anyone who dared think a man who once wore backless pants would care what the public thought of his appearance.

Whether the natural hair movement helped the Black community progress beyond the painful paradigms of "good hair" remains a matter of debate. However, using the Internet to criticize Black hair, whether it was natural or straight, seemed to be a new popular pastime for many in the Black blogosphere and on social media sites. And children weren't safe from the venom.

Black Children's Hair Comes Under Attack

On the evening of August 2, 2012, many Americans sat open-mouthed in front of their televisions, amazed by Olympic gymnast Gabrielle Douglas. After her dizzying routine on the floor, the judges calculated scores while millions continued to marvel over the tiny sixteen-year-old's strength and skill. But a few weren't in awe, they were in attack mode, tweeting messages like "In Olympic news, why hasn't anyone tried to fix Gabby Douglas's hair?" and "Gabby Douglas needs to tame the beady beads in the back of her hair lol." Not surprisingly, gymnasts who spend their time flipping, tumbling, and leaping through the air are not known for having salon-perfect hair. Like Douglas, most launch a bobby pin, hair spray, and gel assault on their buns and ponytails to keep them under some kind of control during competitive matches. The rest of Gabby's teammates' hair did not look much different from hers, yet they did not cause an Internet dust-up. The difference? Douglas is Black, which is why the comments were not contained to a few hateful tweeters.

The day after Gabby won the gold medal, *Daily Beast* ran a quote from a Black woman who said, "I love how she's doing her thing and winning. But I just hate the way her hair looks with all those pins and gel. I wish someone could have helped her make it look better since she's being seen all over the world. She's representing for Black women everywhere." Hairstylist Larry Simms, who works with weave-loving celebs Gabrielle Union and Mary J. Blige, argued, "It's taboo culturally to be seen in public with a kinky hairline and your ponytail is straight. . . . I think Black girls in particular view her as a representation of themselves for the world to see. She just needs some Smooth 'N Shine gel and she'd be okay."

Douglas did not think that she needed anything—after all, she had two gold medals and a permanent spot in Olympic history as the first African-American to win the women's all-around gymnastics title. So in response to the insults she found about her appearance on the Internet, Douglas told the Associated Press, "I don't know where this is coming from. What's wrong with my hair? I just made history and people are focused on my hair? You might as well stop talking about it."

Douglas was right. That should have been the last comment, but a short time later, the public cheered when photos were released of Douglas's brand-new weave, put in by Ted Gibson, stylist and hair makeover maverick of the TV show *What Not to Wear*. "Now that she's got the gold, she's going for the look," said an article on Electronic Urban Report. "Gabby Douglas is getting rid of the bad weave and becoming a real superstar with good hair and all."

The public still had lower to sink, it seemed. Just one year later, in 2013, Beyoncé and Jay Z took their fifteen-month-old daughter to a bistro in Paris for lunch. For one of the most photographed celebrity couples ever, the Carters had made a point to keep their daughter under wraps—literally—taking her out with blankets over her head so the paparazzi could not get a shot. And yet here was Blue Ivy in Paris, playing with her parents as the photos showed her with skinny jeans, a T-shirt, and hair not unlike many babies', meaning it was unstyled, longer on top, and a variety of curl patterns, from loose to tightly coiled. Hours later, as the pictures went viral, critics went into overdrive. A few wanted to know why she was in jeans and a T-shirt instead of a girly dress, but more wanted to lambast Beyoncé, agreeing with celebrity blogger Sandra Rose who wrote, "It's a shame that Beyoncé brought her daughter out in public with her nappy hair looking like Buckwheat. Doesn't Bey carry a comb for such emergencies?"

Author and blogger Denene Millner was outraged by the attacks on an-
other Black child and penned an angry article on her parenting blog
My Brown Baby. To Blue Ivy's critics, Millner wrote, "Leave. That. Baby.
Alone."

In response to the venom spewed in the direction of Blue Ivy, Gabby
and other Black celebrity children, Millner says, "The world is full of key-
board gangsters—people who say some of the ugliest things imaginable
while hiding behind the anonymity of the Internet." She continues,
"[Their] proclamations are steeped in wicked, ridiculous, damaged notions of what Black children's hair should look like—particularly that of
Black girls. I can't help but to think that it's tied into our equally wicked,
ridiculous, damaged notions about Black girls' bodies. We need them to be
tamed. We need them to be restrained. Wild and free and natural is a no-
go. The Internet, then, becomes just another tool in the policeman's arsenal, another way to keep Black girls and Black mothers in our place."

As disgusted as Millner and others were that Blue Ivy would face such
vitriol, this was not the first baby to be publicly ridiculed. That would have
been Zahara Jolie-Pitt, the adopted child of Brad Pitt and Angelina Jolie.
Zahara, who is Ethiopian, was photographed constantly when she was
small and had hair that was apparently so offensive to many that *Newsweek*
reporter Allison Samuels (who is Black herself) wrote an article about it in
2009 headlined "Zahara Jolie-Pitt and the Politics of Uncombed Hair." It
included lines such as "Photos of Zahara show the four-year-old girl sporting hair that is wild and unstyled, uncombed and dry. Basically: a hot
mess. Samuels also wrote, "Not all people will recognize Zahara as the
child of movie royalty. To many, she'll be just a Black little girl—and a
Black girl with bad hair at that."

Despite the fact that criticizing a four-year-old's hair hardly seemed appropriate, Samuels was not alone in her condemnation of Zahara's appearance. Most critics, including Samuels, thought the ones at fault were her
White parents, who did not understand the politics of Black hair in America. And this was despite the fact that Brad Pitt had already gone on record,
when "Z" was just a baby, in an attempt to prove that he knew something
about his daughter's hair.

Brad Pitt shared his hair knowledge with a reporter from *Esquire* magazine in 2006. "For White people who might be having a little trouble with

Black-person hair, Carol's Daughter is a fantastic hair product," he stated. "We got it for Z. Now her hair has this beautiful luster. And it smells nice, too." To some readers it was great that a father was taking an interest in how to do his daughter's hair—especially since her hair is so unlike his own straight, blond mane. But to others, like the thousands of Internet commentators who posted on sites like Crunk + Disorderly and *People* magazine, the actor was completely out of line. How dare Pitt say Black people's hair can be trouble, some asked. How dare he give it another category, "Black-person hair," as if it is not regular hair, others pointed out angrily. Is he implying that normally Black hair doesn't smell nice, unless it has product, others wanted to know.

Mind your own business and stay out of our hair was the general sentiment of his critics, even though it *is* Pitt's business to know how to do his child's hair and to find products that work well for it. By giving his Carol's Daughter endorsement in the pages of *Esquire,* he unwittingly showed that when it comes to Black hair, Black people still want White people to stay silent—since, too often, when they speak, everything goes all wrong.

Black Hair in White Spaces

America was becoming increasingly multicultural in the new millennium, yet there was still a lot of regressive thinking going on about what White people understood and thought about Black hair. The Internet and the increased appearance of Black people on television and in all facets of public life had given White people a lot more opportunity to learn about a topic they may not have known about before. Anyone could see the film *Good Hair* or read an article in *The New York Times* about women transitioning from relaxers to natural. Or, perhaps to the collective embarrassment of the Black community, they could also use the media to follow the Gabby Douglas or Blue Ivy hair controversies. Optimistically, all of this exposure could lead to a better understanding and a new appreciation. And at times it did. Television commercials were increasingly casting natural-haired women, and more fashion magazines were using models with various textures and lengths in beauty shoots. But all too often it led to old-fashioned racism. Even the White House wasn't safe.

By President Barack Obama's second inauguration, the world was in love with Michelle Obama and had declared her a style icon. Two covers of *Vogue* announced her as a fashion world darling, but her hair was also making global news, from blogs to CNN to the BBC. When she got bangs right before the 2013 inauguration—a move that she joked was her "midlife crisis"—the new style was talked about nonstop by the public and press. The First Lady was not exaggerating when she told a Chicago crowd, "My bangs set off a national conversation." *Saturday Night Live* even created a good-natured skit about them.

However, things had not always been so positive when it came to the Obamas and hair. Even before his first election in 2008, Obama and his wife were on the cover of *The New Yorker* in a satirical drawing that showed them depicted as America's worst nightmare. With a flag burning in the fireplace and a framed picture of Bin Laden over the mantel of the Oval Office, Obama stood in Muslim attire giving a fist bump to his wife. Michelle had been outfitted in military gear, with a rifle slung over her shoulder and an Afro to replace her standard straight hairstyle, presumably to up her "scary" quotient. In a throwback to the 1970s, once again the message was that an Afro was militant and hostile and terrifying. And once again, Black people were furious at the implication. New Yorkers of all races were so incensed by the cover that they protested outside of the magazine's offices, led by State Senator Bill Perkins.

As upset as some were about the *New Yorker* cover, it paled greatly to the outrage over Don Imus's attack on Black hair. On April 4, 2007, while discussing the NCAA Women's Basketball Championship, the shock jock host of CBS's *Imus in the Morning* referred to the Rutgers University team, which is made up of eight Black and two White women, as "nappy-headed hos."

Understandably, African-Americans were horrified. The word "nappy" has its roots back in the most violent and racially divided days of the nation's history. When used by White people, it has always demeaned Black people. It was, as the *Today* show said in a story it posted to its Web site about the Imus affair, "the other n-word." Essence Carson, the Rutgers basketball team captain, said his comments had "stolen a moment of pure grace" from the players. Yet at first, Imus insisted he was not the one to blame. The day after the comments, he said, "That phrase [nappy-headed ho] didn't originate in the White community. That phrase originated in the Black community. Young Black women all through that society are demeaned and disparaged and disrespected by their own Black men, and they are called that name in Black hip-hop."

Black people were not willing to take the fall for the vicious words coming out of his mouth. Jesse Jackson called for a boycott, the NAACP demanded his resignation or that the station fire him, and thousands of people—including Oprah Winfrey—did not back down in saying that what he had done was unacceptable. Advertisers were quick to respond and sponsors such as American Express, Sprint, and Staples pulled support from the show. After Al Sharpton called Imus "racist" and "sexist" when he appeared as a guest on Sharpton's show, one week after the initial broadcast, CBS gave in to the mounting pressure and fired Imus.

Post-dismissal, he admitted that what he'd said was unacceptable and he met with the basketball team. The three-hour meeting went well according to the team's coach, and in the following days, Imus acknowledged that his comments were "really stupid."

The same year that Imus was fired, a White *Glamour* magazine editor also lost her job over Black hair. Ashley Baker, a style writer and creator of the Slaves to Fashion blog, was a professional arbiter of fashion dos, don'ts, rights, and wrongs. Baker was invited to Manhattan law firm Cleary Gottlieb to do a presentation on corporate attire and hair. One of her first slides showed an Afro and the quip "Just Say No to the Fro." Though a few women in the audience said they found this offensive, it seemed as if Baker's 'fro faux pas was not a big deal, until the incident was reported weeks later in a law journal. Women's-interest site Jezebel.com covered it in a story titled "Apparently Being Black is Kinda a Corporate Don't." After writing about the Afro slide, they detailed equally disparaging remarks that they claimed Baker made about dredlocs.

Since Jezebel did not name the editor who had done the presentation, Baker was put in the uneasy position of having to out herself in the *Glamour* office, in the midst of reader letters pouring in to express their outrage and disappointment. For six weeks letters came in, the blogosphere went into overdrive detailing the incident, some called for boycotts, and editor-in-chief Cindi Leive went on NPR to discuss what took place. In the end, Baker resigned, Leive issued an apology on the magazine's Web site, and *Glamour* did a three-part series on race, beginning with a roundtable discussion with a multiethnic group of women called "Your Race, Your Looks," a transcript of which ran in the February 2008 issue.

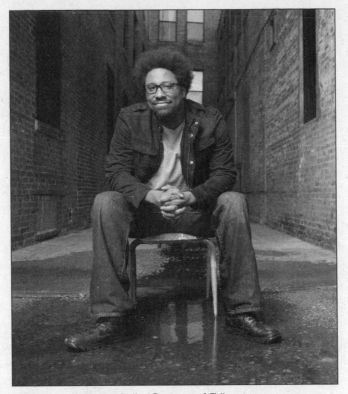

Comedian W. Kamau Bell. (Courtesy of FX)

Baker's biggest offense was not a Don Imus–type of intentional mean-spirited ignorance, but an ignorance of cluelessness. Jezebel columnist Dodai Stewart wrote, "I think that what Ashley Baker has is the luxury of never having been 'other.' She's never probably had to even think about the meaning behind dredlocs or an Afro, so how could she have an informed opinion? The best possible outcome of all this is that she now knows something she didn't know before." Comedian W. Kamau Bell, star of the television show *Totally Biased*, has some general advice for White people when it comes to Black hair that Baker could have used: "Just keep your mouth closed and listen."

After years of being peppered with questions about his own "natural" hair by White people, Bell included a bit about what White people should *never* ask Black people about their hair in his one-man show *The W. Kamau Bell Curve: Ending Racism in About an Hour*. "I don't think we have moved on," he says in explanation of why he included the hair segment. "I think that the nature of the narrative of Black people in this country is so embedded in White America that even 'good' White people still approach you thinking 'I can't own them anymore, but I can ask anything I want.'" That said, Bell cautions, "You can be curious about anything, but that doesn't mean you necessarily get to know the answer."

But not every White person who commented on Black hair got it wrong. In fact, one man got it very right. It all started on *Sesame Street* when a brown Muppet in a pink, puff-sleeved dress and curly Afro came on screen and sang:

"Wear a clippy or a bow or let it sit in an Afro . . . I love my hair, I love my hair, I love it and I have to share. I want to make the world aware I love my hair. I wear it up, I wear it down, I wear it twisted all around. . . ."

The song, called "I Love My Hair," debuted on an episode of *Sesame Street* in October 2010, and its 118 seconds of Black hair adoration became an instant viral sensation. First, excited parents told their friends about it and put the clip on YouTube. Soon, bloggers and users of Facebook and Twitter posted comments and linked to the video online. African-American women wrote that whether or not they had children, the clip made them cry because of its empowering message and its unexpected messenger—namely, *Sesame Street*, more commonly known as the home of Elmo, Cookie Monster, and sing-alongs about numbers, not expressions of Black love and pride.

The praise was so strong and undying that NPR decided to investigate what had prompted *Sesame Street* to enter the Black hair conversation. The answer shocked many: A White man created the clip that had brought so many Black women to tears. Joey Mazzarino, the head writer of *Sesame Street*, wrote the song for his daughter, a five-year-old whom he and his wife adopted from Ethiopia. "She wanted to have long, blond, and straight hair, and she wanted to be able to bounce it around," he told NPR. What surprised Italian-American Mazzarino most was how a song that he hoped would encourage his daughter ended up being embraced by an entire community. Women left comments on the YouTube page, some two years after the clip debuted, with messages such as "I wish I heard this when I was a girl" and "For my black daughter it was inspirational. She smiled and said she loved her hair (after weeks of wanting straight hair); anything helps when you have a toddler trying to see herself as beautiful in the world."

The rest of the mass media and entertainment industry could have

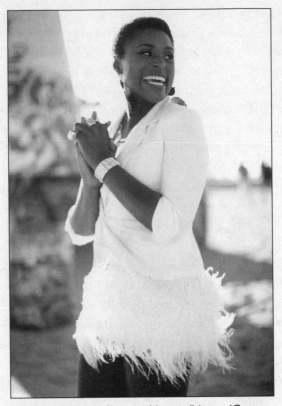

Issa Rae, Hollywood's natural hair trailblazer. (Courtesy of Aspire Network)

benefited from *Sesame Street*'s educated—and positive—approach to Black hair. In Hollywood, long hair and weaves were still the order of the day for Black women. And forget about reality television—with its dizzying revolving door of weaves, wigs, and add-ons, it was one of the most unlikely places to find real hair on a Black female character.

Actresses did not fare much better. Halle Berry was one of the few exceptions of a Black actress with short hair, yet was frequently in movie roles wearing a wig or weave. Kerry Washington, star of the ABC show *Scandal*, had natural hair but it was altered (and lengthened) for her on-screen appearances. When Viola Davis showed up at the 2012 Academy Awards, more shocking than the fact that a Black woman had been nominated for Best Actress was that she was at the ceremony with a short Afro. Davis made headlines for leaving her wig at home. And while everyone

applauded her look—including the natural hair community, *InStyle* magazine, and even the brutally sarcastic hosts of E!'s *Fashion Police* TV show—
over a year later she still had not been seen with natural hair on-screen.

Issa Rae, twenty-nine, was looking to change that. While she was not
focused specifically on Viola Davis, Rae wanted it to be normal for various
textures of Black hair to be a common sight on screens large and small.
Rae's Web series *The Misadventures of Awkward Black Girl*, a comedy about
the life of a socially awkward African-American woman named Jay, brought
her to national attention and eventually led to a talk show and her own series on HBO. Though that alone made Rae a groundbreaking maverick, so,
too, did her approach to hair. In an industry of long and flowing, she was
short and natural. So was *Awkward*'s Jay, played by Rae and subjected to a
long-running subplot that her short hair must mean that she is a lesbian,
even though she is in a relationship with a man. Jay's hair was just the first
step in presenting alternative images to what Rae called "Hollywood hair,"
which she says was based on European standards. "While I am happy with
how as a community Black people are embracing our [natural] hair, I hope
that Hollywood catches up," she says. "And I hope to have a part in changing and opening the limiting images that we see."

Black Hair's Promising Future

With hair renegades like Rae making inroads in Hollywood, and real
women everywhere wearing Afros, locs, braids, wigs, weaves, perms, and
whatever else, in many ways the early twenty-first century was an aesthetic free-for-all. Films like 2002's *Barbershop*, Willow Smith's 2010 hair
anthem and girl-power video "I Whip My Hair Back and Forth," books
like the always-popular Nappily Ever After series by Trisha R. Thomas,
documentaries like 2012's *In Our Heads About Our Hair*, and the art work of
painters like Tim Okamura and photographer Nakeya Brown showed that
cultural productions were also exploring and celebrating Black hair and
Black hair culture.

Unfortunately, alongside these positives were the continued attacks
against Black hair. They included the letter sent home to parents by an
Ohio school in 2013 saying that Afro puffs and small twists were banned in
the high school as part of a strict new dress code intended to foster a

"successful school environment." And these attacks also provoked discrimination lawsuits being brought against Federal Express, Disney, and Six Flags for refusing employment to Black people because of their hairstyles. It was a sad repeat of cases that plagued the tourism industry in the 1980s.

And while America continued to grapple with its tangled Black hair history, the rest of the world was joining the conversation. In the last years of the Divided Decade, natural hair conventions had taken place in London, Paris, Madrid, and throughout cities in Europe with sizable Black populations. May 18, 2013, was declared International Natural Hair Meetup Day and on that spring day, there were gatherings in cities all over the United States as well as in the Netherlands and Japan. Celebrity natural-hair stylist Felicia Leatherwood even took her Loving Your Hair with Natural Care workshop to sold-out venues in Germany and Senegal.

In Latin America, where the phrase *"pelo bueno, pelo malo,"* (good hair, bad hair) was coined, a natural hair consciousness movement was also under way. This was exemplified through the work of women such as Carolina Contreras and Tasmy Gomez, Dominican women who led natural hair workshops and spread their gospel on their Web site Missrizos.com. Meanwhile, in Puerto Rico, Joaquin Medina and Kali Blocker launched their Diosas al Natural (natural goddesses) organization that promoted *el orgullo* (pride) in non-straight textures. "As a community—especially where we are at in this wonderful moment of really being seen and embracing each other as a truly diverse tribe—we prize authenticity over both trends and traditions," says author and editor Veronica Chambers, who considers herself an "outlier" as a Black Latina with dredlocs. "In that way, there's room for all kinds of Latina hair stories to be told in the years ahead."

Perhaps it all goes back to what many therapists, natural hair bloggers, salon owners, and wise mothers say—you need to talk about something to get to the other side. And Americans had never talked as much, or as honestly, about Black hair as they did during this era. The question is: What will the conversation be for the next generation, who was raised on the Internet, exposed to increased multiculturalism, and is able to enjoy a growing familiarity with natural hair textures? Guaranteed, Black hair will remain a dynamic topic rooted in love, pride, and identity.

The "Dramatic Potential" in Black Hair: A Q&A with Author Chimamanda Ngozi Adichie

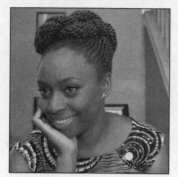

Chimamamanda Ngozi Adichie
(Courtesy of Ivara Esege)

Chimamanda Ngozi Adichie is an award-winning Nigerian novelist who splits her time between the United States and Nigeria. Her fiction deftly explores life in Nigeria before, after, and during the Biafran war. But in her 2013 novel, *Americanah,* Adichie sets her story in several major U.S. cities, as well as Lagos and London. It's a modern-day tale about life, love . . . and Black hair.

In *Americanah,* the protagonist, a Nigerian woman living in the United States, spends a lot of time thinking about her hair. Do you spend a lot of time thinking about your hair?

Not as much as I used to. Or maybe I still do but in a different way. Before I worried about my hair. Now I find much pleasure in hair thoughts. When I first went natural, I was obsessed with thoughts of what to "do" to my hair. It was a problem to solve. Now that I have fallen in love with my hair, I am much more sanguine.

Has #teamnatural made its way to Nigeria?

The idea of wearing natural hair as a choice is still very young in Nigeria. But the natural hair movement *is* growing. It started, I think, with Nigerians who had lived in the U.S.

But the [hairdressers] still have no idea how to take care of natural hair. In general I choose to wash my hair myself, but the few times I do go to a salon in Lagos, I am always in gentle and not-so-gentle negotiations with the hairdressers. "Don't put that comb in my hair while it's so dry and tangled! Don't use that small comb! No! Untangle it with your fingers! Be gentle! Divide it into sections first!" And on and on. Sadly, many hairdressers are much better at taking care of weaves than they are of actual hair, whether relaxed or natural.

Does Black hair culture in the United States make for good material as a novelist?

Yes. Specifically Black women's hair. The way hair often comes loaded with assumptions—how some people, for example, think a woman wearing dredlocs is somehow more "authentic" or "soulful." And especially now with this growing movement of Black women learning to love their [natural] look, it's a new subculture that has a lot of dramatic potential.

You've admitted publicly that you're easily distracted by natural hair videos on YouTube. What's the fascination?
I am simply fascinated by this subculture of Black women's hair, how transnational it is with vloggers from the U.S. and the Caribbean and the UK, and how the conversation is so much more than just about hair. It says something about confidence and a new and wonderful sense of self.

Over the course of your literary career, your hairstyles have changed dramatically. Does your hairstyle say something about where you are in your creative process as a writer?
No, it says a lot more about where I am in my growth process as a woman.

I used to love long extension braids. Now I'm indifferent to them. I used to wear curly weaves, because I thought they were "mainstream" enough, while not being too far from my true aesthetic. But I didn't actually like the tight feeling of weaves, the ickiness after I worked out, or the lack of full access to my scalp. Then I decided to go closer to my true aesthetic. And for me, my true aesthetic is: How do I wear my hair in a way that makes me feel most like myself? Now I wear cornrows with just my hair. I roll and pin my hair. I try African threading styles. It's still very much in progress but I feel most like myself when I am wearing just my hair, no extensions, in a style that I think is beautiful.

The Business of Black Hair 2.0

In 2001, Jamyla Bennu was a Brooklyn-based freelancer, earning a modest living from a host of creative jobs that ranged from Web site design to dancing. A self-described "crafty person," when she couldn't find the perfect products for her naturally kinky hair, Bennu decided to make them herself, following recipes that called for everyday ingredients she could easily find at the grocery store. Excited by the process, Bennu didn't stop with hair products. She taught herself to make bath and body products as well and soon started gifting them to friends and family. It wasn't long before she was selling her homemade concoctions at holiday and craft fairs to augment her freelance income. In 2003, using what back then were considered highly specialized skills, Bennu created a Web site so she could sell her products to a wider audience, especially to all of the virtual friends she'd met on online forums dedicated to natural hair maintenance. She dubbed her fledgling company Oyin Handmade. Oyin means "honey" in Yoruba, and it is one of the central ingredients in many of her products. "It was the beginning of e-commerce," Bennu says, laughing now at her humble beginnings. "It was just me in my kitchen, but the Web site gave me instant professionalism."

By 2005, Bennu and her husband, Pierre, also a creative freelancer, realized that Bennu's little hair business wasn't so little. "At first Oyin was just one of many things we were doing to make money," recalls Bennu. "Then all of a sudden it was all we were doing." Taking a leap of faith, the couple left Brooklyn and bought a house in Baltimore that was big enough to establish Oyin's base of operations in the basement. Today, Oyin Handmade operates out of a commercial space in Baltimore and employs eleven people including Bennu, now thirty-seven, and her husband. Annual revenue in 2012 was $750,000, and 2014 will be the year when they see their products sold nationwide on the shelves of a major chain retailer.

Oyin Handmade is no overnight success story; it was over ten years in the making, yet one can't help but be inspired by the narrative of a young Black woman providing homemade quality hair products to a neglected consumer, providing jobs to people in her community, and profiting financially. Not only is the story inspirational, it's also a bit familiar.

The beginning of the twenty-first century in the Black hair care industry feels eerily like a rerun of the twentieth century. One could simply substitute Bennu's story for Madam C. J. Walker's or Annie Turnbo Malone's. A Black woman of modest means, frustrated by the lack of products in the marketplace made for her hair, watches her homemade creations become beauty must-haves for thousands of women previously ignored by the mainstream beauty industry. Memorialized today as revolutionaries in the Black hair care industry, Walker and Malone had no background in either business or cosmetology—coincidentally, neither did Bennu, whose degree is in philosophy—they just wanted a source of income and a beautiful, healthy head of hair. Yet they were beloved by their customers and championed by the Black community; their success shed a positive light on Black entrepreneurship and more importantly, provided Black women—and quite a few men—the products and permission to be beautiful.

Fast-forward to the middle of the 1900s, however, when the success of the Black hair business caused White-owned companies to wake up and take action. Through trial and error and then just plain acquisitions and mimicry, the end of the twentieth century witnessed an almost complete takeover of Black-owned hair-care companies by large White-owned conglomerates. So, will history repeat itself? Will the twenty-first century experience the same unhappy ending?

The New Normal: Naturals

One of the biggest changes to affect the ethnic hair industry in the first decade of the twenty-first century was the shift Black women made from relaxed to natural hairstyles. The shift started slowly enough, but by 2008, what had been a subtle change had turned into an obvious trend—and it was affecting the bottom line for those who profited from Black women's love of bone-straight tresses. Industry insiders predicted a continuous 23 percent decline in relaxer sales through the year 2011. Partly, that fall-off was due to the recession that hit that same year, causing some women to give up their relaxers simply to save money. But for many, it was just time to reconnect with their roots. "People were becoming more in touch with what is true and real in life," says Anu Prestonia, owner of Khamit Kinks natural hair salon in New York City. "I think we were just moving towards an age of enlightenment," she adds. Regardless of the reason, there was no denying that natural was fast becoming the new normal.

The Jheri Curl-ization of the Natural Hair Movement

Back in the 1960s and 70s, when the Back to Natural movement took hold of Black America, the hair-care industry came to a standstill, and many lost their jobs. Why? Because an Afro required little maintenance and few products. Salon owners, product manufacturers, and beauty supply distributors considered the natural look to be a natural disaster. But not this time. The new natural hair movement inspired a veritable orgy of product development, heretofore unseen since the drippy and immensely profitable days of the Jheri Curl. From curl creams to scalp serums, the beauty industry quickly found ways to capitalize on the desires of the new naturalistas to have long, thick, healthy hair. And this wasn't just a trend in ethnic hair care. Market research projected that the overall organic hair and body product sectors would surpass $13 billion in sales by 2016. Very quickly, it seemed, the natural hair movement was being commercialized in such a way that a multitude of products had to be purchased in order to maintain the natural look. No longer would a good jar of grease and an Afro pick suffice.

Mainstream manufacturers, witnessing the introduction of natural hair products in the marketplace by mostly Black female entrepreneurs, responded by taking their already existing products and changing the packaging, perhaps adding some exotic-sounding oils or fruit juices to their shampoos and conditioners. A stroll down the hair products aisle at the local drugstore suddenly felt like a walk in the supermarket on a Caribbean island. Coconuts, mangos, and avocados graced the labels of bottles that were now brown, green, and beige instead of fluorescent pinks and yellows. Procter & Gamble, for example, tried to appeal to the new naturalistas without alienating their core consumers by calling their "new" Pantene hair-care line Relaxed and Natural. And the bottles were switched from white to brown. But the savvy Black female consumer wasn't so easily convinced that these newly "natural" mainstream products were her best option.

Armed with the knowledge gleaned from Web sites, blogs, and online forums, not only was she aware of the products on the market that didn't live up to their hype—or worse, those that could actually cause her hair damage—she also had access to products, like Oyin Homemade or Karen's Body Beautiful, that were being produced in small batches and distributed online or at street fairs or even out of someone's home. Indeed, the consumer demand for products specifically made for natural hair by trustworthy manufacturers inspired many folks to jump into the hair-care game.

Biracial women were some of the first success stories in the game. Having struggled for years to find mainstream products that catered to their unique—often curly but not quite kinky—hair, they too started creating products and forming successful hair-care companies. Companies like Mixed Chicks and Miss Jessie's were some of the first curly hair products on mainstream store shelves, including Target and Duane Reade, paving the way for products made specifically for Black natural hair. And while women of mixed racial heritage created those companies with multiracial hair in mind, Black women who embraced their natural hair championed their message, which is namely to love their curls.

But not every new "naturalpreneur" was a neophyte in the beauty business. Jane Carter came to the table armed with more than a decade of experience and education in the hair industry. Carter was a successful and popular stylist and salon owner in New Jersey, always working with clients of different ethnic backgrounds and hair types. In 1992 she started experiencing allergy symptoms in response to some of the chemicals in the products she was using in her salon. In short order she threw out all of the products that were making her ill, signed up for a course on essential oils, and created her first 100-percent natural hair product, Hair Nourishing Serum, to use in her salon. Soon enough her clients,

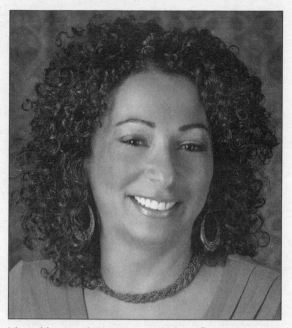

Natural hair product entrepreneur Jane Carter. (Courtesy Allison V. Brown)

both Black and White, wanted to buy it and an idea for a company was born.

"The entrepreneurial spirit is part of my DNA," says the mother of two. By 2005, sales of her products were doing so well, Carter sold her salon in order to focus solely on the growth of what she officially dubbed The Jane Carter Solution. By 2007, the company, based in East Orange, New Jersey, posted $1.7 million in sales. Today Carter is the CEO and chief chemist of The Jane Carter Solution, and her all-natural hair products for all textures can be purchased at such diverse retailers as Whole Food Markets and Target, as well as online. "My expertise in the beauty business is our company's greatest strength," says Carter, who continues to create new products for her brand. "I know how a product has to perform because I have all this insight from working in this business for so long."

Natural Hair Means Big Business

Needless to say, these women who engaged in natural hair product manufacturing weren't the only ones making money from the natural hair trend.

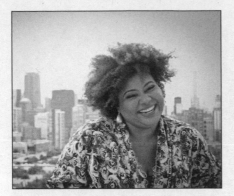

The beautiful face behind Afrobella, Patrice Yursik. (Courtesy of Chuck Olu-Alabi)

A cottage industry that included bloggers, authors, event planners, salon owners, and even jewelry and T-shirt designers sprouted up as people from all walks of life realized there was money to be made from natural hair. Even people with no previous hair experience found a way to make a profit and sometimes earn a living from the natural hair mania sweeping the country.

Patrice Yursik, thirty-four, was the assistant calendar editor of the alternative weekly *The Miami New Times* when she started a blog called Afrobella in 2006. With dreams of being a fiction writer, Yursik used her blog simply as an outlet to share her opinions and ideas about beauty from a more diverse perspective than what she could find in the mainstream press. "I wanted it to be like the magazine I couldn't find on the newsstand," says the Trinidadian native. Her first post was about her own natural hair journey; her second explored how Josephine Baker was a style icon. She obviously hit a nerve because soon enough her work as a blogger was getting her more attention than her job at the newspaper.

Today Afrobella is Yursik's full-time job, and she's making more money than she did as an assistant editor, but she admits it's taken her a long time and a lot of work to get there. Often referred to as the "godmother of brown beauty blogging," Yursik spends her days blogging, speaking, tweeting, acting as a spokesperson, and literally traveling around the world attending events often centered on the world of natural hair. By 2013, she had over 45,000 followers on Twitter, and *Ebony* magazine added her to their Power 100 list in 2011, which also included President Barack Obama and Oprah Winfrey. Yursik knows she's in an enviable position, and she knows many people have tried to copy her success. A search on Google for "Black hair blogs" brings up close to 300 million results. "The blogosphere has gotten a little redundant," says Yursik. "But there are always new platforms to explore. The next Afrobella might be on YouTube."

Alicia Nicole Walton, thirty, isn't trying to be the next Afrobella, because she's already staked her claim in the natural hair blogosphere. Known online as Curly Nikki, Walton brings new meaning to the idea of a natural hair entrepreneur. A licensed psychotherapist originally from St. Louis, Missouri, Walton started blogging in 2008 after building up a loyal following on the Web site NaturallyCurly.com. She rose to fame not only by sharing her thoughts on different products and talking about her latest hairstyles, but also by paying attention to the emotional and psychological issues involved with making the lifestyle change required in going natural. It seems like an obvious connection given her background in psychology. And then of course there is Walton's personality. Even though she's addressing thousands of women on her blog, readers get the impression that her straight talk is only being shared with her BFFs, be it about a recent hair-related drugstore discovery, or the latest shenanigans of her young daughter.

"She's a star," says Michelle Breyer, president of Textured Media, the umbrella company that purchased the CurlyNikki Web site for a substantial but undisclosed sum in 2009. "She's a hair icon, a fashion icon, a mom icon." And as an icon, Walton has seen the financial results of her online success. In addition to the sale of her Web site and a percentage from the advertisements running on CurlyNikki.com, Walton continues to find new ways to profit from her natural hair knowledge. "I've successfully secured several six-figure contracts and developed new revenue streams," she says, including writing the 2013 bestselling book *Better Than Good Hair* and creating the CurlyNikki meetups. They are more than a gathering of women gabbing about their hair, Walton says, "In 2010, I took [the meetup] concept and totally *fabbed* it out by conducting brand-sponsored and totally free soirées all over the country." In other words, a CurlyNikki meetup is paid for by corporate brands that want to bank on Walton's popularity and ability to draw a crowd. Walton's meetups, which have even occurred overseas, receive thousands of RSVPs from women eager to share and learn about new products and new styles. "I'm proud to see that this model has caught on and that natural hair meetups are now just as prevalent—perhaps even more so—as hair shows," Walton says.

Walton and Yursik certainly aren't the only bloggers to earn a living or at least a decent amount of pocket change by offering information, product reviews, and a space to vent about their hair in a supportive community. The frequency with which Black women were making money by blogging and creating YouTube tutorials on natural hair styles and maintenance was so great that *The New York Times* featured an article about the trend in 2011 with the headline "Going Natural' Requires Lots of Help." Within that story, *Times* reporter Jamila Bey also indicated that the growing popularity of hair shows geared specifically toward the natural hair community was another indicator of the strength of this new natural economy. If you build it—and "it" is natural hair—they will come, seemed to be the name of the game. And that's exactly what Celena McAfee learned in 2013.

McAfee, forty-four, is a graphic designer born and raised in Philadelphia. She is neither a professional hair stylist nor does she have a reputation in the natural hair community. Like most "naturalpreneurs," McAfee found inspiration in her own hair story. McAfee decided to stop relaxing her hair and went natural in 2009. Because she didn't consult a professional, the results were disastrous and required a lot of trial and error until she figured out how to successfully manage and style her hair. Predictably, she started a blog to chart her progress, and that's when she realized she wanted to help other women get the kind of information she wished she'd had during her journey. Enlisting the help of her friend, Monique Eversley, a freelance event planner, the two decided to host a natural hair show in Philadelphia, a city known for its weave and wig lovers. McAfee says her number-one financial goal for the show was to simply stay out of debt. She needed to attract 500 attendees in order to break even on her investment. Instead, McAfee was floored when over twice that number lined up on the day of the event, held in a Sheraton Hotel in downtown Philadelphia in May 2013. "We had more than thirteen hundred people," MacAfee says, still stunned by the turnout. "I think it shows that people are hungry for this information."

The professional hair community needed information about natural hair as well. Because Black women who were choosing to go natural often couldn't find an informed hairdresser, celebrity stylist Anthony Dickey decided to do something about it. The Seattle-born, New York City–based visionary behind the Hair Rules brand and salon says he wrote his book *Hair Rules!: The Ultimate Hair-Care Guide for Women with Kinky, Curly, or Wavy Hair* in 2003 partly because he was dismayed by the lack of knowledge both consumers *and* stylists had about working with textured hair. "I wanted to provide information to level the playing field," says Dickey. Following the success of the book and the subsequent browning of his formerly mostly White clientele, Dickey created his Hair Rules product line meant for all different hair textures, from extremely kinky to perfectly straight. "If it wasn't going to be about knowledge and have a textural specific approach, then it would just be another product line," Dickey says about the standards he set for himself. "Most women who were going natural put too much stock in the products but didn't have enough information," he adds. The Hair Rules line—which debuted in 2008—stands out in the marketplace because most of the products come with online video tutorials that actually show customers how to properly apply and use the products.

Dickey was clearly taking advantage of online communication to reach his consumers and he, as well as others, points to the proliferation of Internet communication as a major driving force in the consumer push for more and better products made for natural Black hair. By sharing information online, consumers can make or break a product. Or at the very least they can get manufacturers to take notice of their dissatisfaction. That's what occurred with the Dr. Miracle's brand. Many natural hair bloggers, including Yursik of Afrobella, refused to try the company's products because of what they considered an offensive and regressive advertising campaign—one that featured before and after shots of a Black woman who looked like she'd been struck by lightning until she used the Dr. Miracle's product. Some bloggers also criticized the fact that the company did not list their product ingredients anywhere on the packaging. The company took note; the offensive commercials ceased, ingredients were listed on some (not all) of the products, and the entire Dr. Miracle's product line was re-launched in 2011. Dozens of natural hair bloggers were on the launch party guest list.

Manufacturers who wanted to stay in business had to listen to this more educated consumer as well as to the bloggers who had become the new arbiters of style, product efficacy, and hair-care regimens in this increasingly natural world. In fact, many Black hair-care manufacturers have trimmed their traditional advertising budgets, choosing to spend money on courting these influential bloggers instead of paying for ad space in magazines, newspapers, or on television. Some of the newcomers on the scene—like Jane Carter—have eschewed traditional advertising altogether and opt for a strategy of social media saturation, free sampling, and plain old word of mouth. "I'd rather put products in people's hands," says Carter, who says she sends thousands of free samples to events and bloggers annually.

Stylists, too, have to be mindful of the influence of natural hair bloggers. "People were visiting YouTube, and the salon became the enemy," says Khamit Kinks owner Anu Prestonia about the early days of the natural hair movement. "I heard so many women on social media say, 'I'm so glad

I went natural so I don't have to go to the salon anymore.'" Eventually, her customers came back and new naturalistas joined them once women realized that the salons are where the professionals are—and cyberspace isn't. "I'm seeing a lot of damaged hair from people trying a million and one things from YouTube and having a closet full of products," says Prestonia.

YouTube wasn't the only challenge for professional stylists. Black hair salons had to deal with some significant industry changes in the first decade of the twenty-first century. For salons that specialized in braiding, new state laws were enacted that required stylists to log over one thousand hours of cosmetology training—training that often had nothing to do with braiding—in order to stay in business. Coupled with the recession and the dip in women choosing to relax their hair, hundreds of African-American salons across the country closed between 2008 and 2010. But not every Black salon lost customers during these turbulent times. In certain parts of the U.S., Black-owned barbershops and salons actually experienced steady if not improved business throughout the recession. One example, in Prince George's County, Maryland, where more than half of the population is African-American, the number of beauty salons and hair stylists increased by 10 percent between 2008 and 2009. This jump gave credence to the myth that the Black hair-care industry is recession-proof. One explanation economists give for this trend is that when people are out of work and regularly going on job interviews, appearance is especially important, so hair salons will stay busy.

Of course, the salons and stylists that rode out the recession with the most success were the ones who were able to keep up with the trends. This included working with natural hair, incorporating new treatments like the Brazilian keratin treatment into their repertoire, and getting comfortable working with extensions and weaves. In fact, any stylist who shifted her focus to weaves during this decade was sure to make a profit.

Still Un-Beweavable

On a Friday morning in the Germantown section of Philadelphia, business is booming at The Weave Bar. Sandwiched between a check-cashing joint and a sneaker store, The Weave Bar sits above the fray. Not only because it's located on the second floor of a nondescript two-story building, away from the noise of the busy street below, but also because The Weave Bar elevates the

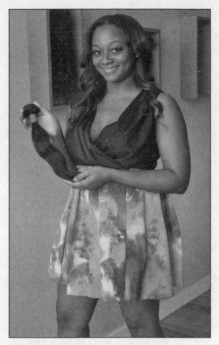

Yolanda Bailey of the Weave Bar.
(Courtesy of Yolanda Bailey)

experience of getting a weave to a streamlined and efficient operation.

Customers enter The Weave Bar, fill out a menu card, and are immediately ushered to one of thirteen chairs in the modern yet minimalist salon with exposed brick accent walls and a shiny hardwood floor. Only a couple of seats are open, and it's just 10:30 in the morning. The allure is simple: For fifty dollars, a patron can get a signature sew-in weave and be out of the chair in less than two hours. (The average cost for a weave is $150.) They can also choose from a posted menu of à la carte services, such as detail cuts, color, or a flat iron, depending on their needs. If getting a weave at The Weave Bar feels slightly like a fast-food experience—"you're in, you order, you're out"—then that's a good thing. "The average time at a traditional salon is four hours," explains Weave Bar co-owner and manager, Yolanda Bailey, thirty-one. "We shaved that by half. That's our secret sauce," she quips. "We do à la carte services as well so women can decide for themselves, 'I want this instead of that.'"

Clearly her Burger King "I'll have my weave my way" system is working. Bailey and her husband opened their first Weave Bar in West Philadelphia in 2012. One year later, they opened the Germantown salon, followed quickly by the opening of a retail store called Pink Label Beauty, where they sell their own private-label hair extensions and hair products. Given that The Weave Bar in Germantown often has a line out the door on Saturday mornings, Bailey is far from done with expanding her brand. "We're looking for a third location," she admits, amazed at the runaway success of her fledgling company.

Yes, it may seem paradoxical that when the entire country had embraced the idea of "natural," more and more women were opting for fake hair. But the numbers don't lie. Despite the decline in relaxer sales and the obvious boom in organic and natural hair products, the percentage of Black women who continued to wear their hair in a straightened style, using either chemicals, extreme heat, or an add-on product like a wig or a weave, remained significant throughout the first thirteen years of the new millennium. In fact, during this divided decade, more than 70 percent of Black women still chose chemically straightened hair over wearing their natural locs. And Yolanda Bailey estimates that 50 to 60 percent of her weave customers have natural hair under their weaves, begging the question of what "going natural" really means. As a businessperson in the add-on hair industry, it simply means the market is wide open.

By the end of the twentieth century, many Black movie stars, models, and celebrities regularly wore wigs and weaves, but the common person did not. In the twenty-first century, things changed. Diane Da Costa, owner of Simplee Beautiful Salon in Westchester, New York, says there's a reason beyond trendiness why weaves increased in popularity: They have been upgraded in quality and versatility. "In the past, weaves only came in two textures: silky waves and straight," she says. "Now extension hair is available in all textures and includes straight, waves, curly, very curly, and even highly textured, tight, coily hair. This is a major difference because it doesn't look fake or like you're trying to be someone you're not." Da Costa also notes that the technology associated with applying weaves has improved such that it's much harder to tell when someone is wearing one. With that kind of versatility and quality, the weave industry flourished, as more and more people beyond the celebrity set experimented with them.

Even after Chris Rock's revelatory *Good Hair* ripped the curtain off the gritty reality involved in collecting human hair from India—where the United States imports the greatest amount of human hair—the industry didn't come to a standstill. On the contrary, it continues to grow, supported not only by Black women, but also by significant numbers of White women.

This burgeoning demand for hair extensions has inspired a very brisk business in the sale of human hair, specifically Remy hair. Considered the gold standard in human hair, Remy hair (alternatively spelled Remi) garners a lot of hype, when it actually only means that the hair was shorn from one single (human) head and kept in the same direction, roots to tip, Scott Carney an investigative reporter and author of an award-winning book on the illegal trade of human body parts, was researching the hair trade in India in 2010. He expected to find an unscrupulous industry, but he did not. "The market didn't seem so bad," Carney says, noting that the majority of Remy hair comes from the numerous temples across the country that collect hair as a form of religious sacrifice. "I did not feel that there was any undue exploitation in it." The temples sell the hair directly to the hair traders and use the money for their cause. "When I asked the [Indian people] what they thought about it, they were happy the temples were making money from [the hair]."

On the other hand, Carney did admit that the process of collecting human hair can just be plain gross. "Human hair contains all sorts of secretions, including sweat and blood, plus food particles, lice, and the coconut oil many Indians use as conditioner," he wrote in a subsequent article on the hair industry for *Mother Jones* magazine. In addition, Carney notes that it's only Remy hair that comes from the temple sacrifices. "If it doesn't say Remy, it comes from garbage cans," he says, adding that there are some in India who earn money by going door-to-door collecting hair from women's combs or off the floor of barbershops or even, he says, by digging through garbage cans.

The worldwide demand is so great for Indian hair that a kilo (that's 2.2 pounds) of the raw product can sell for nearly $200 at auction to traders who will then sell it to foreign markets—the top three markets being the United States, China, and the United Kingdom—for a handsome profit. Once that hair makes it to the United States, it will be packaged and sold to stylists and to consumers at prices that frequently have been marked up over 100 percent. The price for a three-ounce package of Remy hair can range from $75 to $200. Most women will need two packages for a single style. And that's just for the hair itself; it doesn't include the stylist's fee or the weekly maintenance required to keep it looking good. Weave maintenance averages around $400 a month. So the stylists who specialize in weaves and the shopkeepers who sell the hair are making a killing. "The average stylist in Philadelphia makes $22,000 a year," says Bailey of The Weave Bar. "My stylists earn twice that much."

And it's not just weaves that have changed the add-on hair game. In the last ten years, wigs have become popular for the mainstream consumer. Where wigs used to be considered appropriate only for Black women of a certain age, thanks to celebrities like rapper Nicki Minaj and talk-show host Wendy Williams, wigs have become high-concept fashion accessories. And like the twenty-first-century weaves, the twenty-first-century wig is a whole new way to have the hair you always wanted.

The new millennium excitement in the wig business has centered on the lace-front wig. Worn by men and women—including celebrities like Beyoncé, Tyra Banks, and even natural hair enthusiast and singer Jill Scott—the genius behind the lace-front wig is the almost imperceptible flesh-colored lace cap. Depending on how much money a patron wants to spend, the lace cap is custom cut (and sometimes custom dyed to match the skin color) to the shape of the person's head and then glued or pinned in place. Because of the delicate lace, a person can part their hair, run their fingers through it and even show off their hairline, tricks previously unheard of with a wig. What's more, these hardy wigs can be worn for weeks at a time and can be shampooed, swam, and slept in. It's like having a hair transplant that simply needs updating every three months. And how much does one of these wonder wigs cost? Celebrities wanting a custom-made lace-front wig made from 100-percent Remy hair can expect to pay nearly $20,000 per wig. Custom wigs with Remy hair for noncelebrities range between $400 and $1,500. Either way, it can be a very lucrative business as more people embrace the flexibility and versatility of a wig. In fact, celebrities like Williams, talk-show personality Sherri Shepherd, and actress Vivica A. Fox aren't just known for wearing wigs, they sell them too, offering fans the opportunity to literally copy their hairstyle.

Not surprisingly, as weaves and wigs become more popular, with limited supply, increasing demand and exorbitant prices of human hair, a criminal element has spread throughout the industry. From South Africa to India there have been reports of women (and men) with long hair being attacked on the streets, in movie theaters, and even in their own homes by thieves who chop off their hair to sell on the black market. In 2004, Britain's *Guardian* newspaper uncovered the disturbing fact that the human hair exported from Russia—used primarily for White women's extensions—most likely came from the shaving of female "prisoners, mental patients, and children against their will." Like the United Kingdom, the United States doesn't have strong regulations in place over human hair imports. In fact, according to official records from the Office of the United States Trade Representative, the United States didn't import any hair from Peru or Malaysia in the last five years, yet several American weave shops claim to be selling it. So that 100-percent Peruvian hair may not really be human, it may have entered the United States in an illegal fashion, or it may just be really old.

There's no denying that a bustling black market for human hair exists all over the world. It remains to be seen whether the U.S. government will get involved. The government has no choice but to get involved, though, in the trend of increasingly bold thieves targeting beauty supply stores and hair salons. But they're not after money; they just want the hair.

In May 2011, *The New York Times* reported on a disturbing new crime spree. Thieves were breaking into beauty supply stores, wig shops, and salons and stealing thousands of dollars' worth of weave hair. And most often, they only took the good stuff. "Whoever did it knew exactly what they wanted," salon owner Lisa Amosu told the *Times*. The criminals stole $150,000 worth of human hair from Amosu's Houston-based salon, My Trendy Place. "They didn't even bother with the synthetic hair," Amosu added. These hair thefts were taking place all over the country, from Texas to Chicago, and the stolen goods would show up as hot product on the Black hair black market, selling to unscrupulous stylists, customers looking for a discount, and ironically, back to the original store owners who had been robbed. A Michigan man, Jay Shin, lost his life in such a robbery in March of 2011. One sobering news headline declared "Beauty Supply Owner Killed Over Six Bags of Hair."

Black Hair, White Hands?

In April 2009, the Black hair care industry came back to Black. The legendary hair-care company Johnson Products hadn't had a Black owner since 1993. In an event reminiscent of a Hollywood revenge film, husband and wife team Eric Brown and Renee Cottrell-Brown, with the backing of two private-equity investment firms, spearheaded an attempt to purchase Johnson Products from Procter & Gamble. The buyback was reportedly a $30-million-dollar purchase.

As the makers of the Ultra Sheen brand of relaxers and hair products, Johnson Products was grossing more than $20 million at the time of sale, according to reports. Many in the industry saw this buyback as more than a good business deal; it was payback. It was an opportunity for Black people to be in charge of one of their own most iconic brands again, and Brown and Cottrell-Brown seemed up to the challenge. Renee Cottrell-Brown was the daughter of Black hair royalty. Her father, Comer Cottrell, founded Pro-Line Corp., makers of the wildly famous 1980s at-home curly perm, the Curly Kit. Cottrell-Brown and her husband had both held high-level positions at Pro-Line, so they knew what to expect and how to prepare. Eric

Brown made a statement about their plans for Johnson Products after the sale went through. "The new Johnson Products Company will provide us with a platform to bring product innovations and promotions to a unique multicultural consumer group and reintroduce the brands to a new generation."

But those plans never got a chance to materialize. In February 2013 Johnson Products Company was sold to Dr. Miracle's, an ethnic hair-care company owned by a private equity firm. A company spokesperson for the newly titled DRMJPC company rationalized the merger this way: "[It] allows the company to now address a larger demographic that crosses generations of African-American women through its updated brand portfolio." Meanwhile, Brown and Cottrell-Brown are no longer with the company.

For many, the story of Johnson Products being swallowed up by a decidedly lesser-known White-owned corporate entity is a portent of what's to come for the few remaining Black-owned manufacturers of Black hair products. It's a trend that started as soon as Madam Walker and Annie Malone made their first million, and it is a trend that will likely continue as long as the ethnic hair-care business remains a $9 billion industry.

But not everyone in the business is bemoaning White investment in Black hair care.

Lisa Price, the founder and president of Carol's Daughter products, is a businesswoman at heart and bristles at the notion that she or anybody else who starts a small business should eschew the investment dollars of non-Blacks. "In general, business success is defined by a smaller company being purchased by a larger entity," she says. Adding that the concern over whether the investor is Black or White is really irrelevant. "If it's the right investor, it's the right investor," she says. And Carol's Daughter has indeed attracted some high-profile investors, both Black and White. In 2005, in a widely publicized deal, a group of celebrities that included Jada Pinkett-Smith, Will Smith, Mary J. Blige, and Jay Z invested $10 million in the brand. The deal was arranged by music exec–turned–marketing specialist Steve Stoute, who had become Price's business partner. And then two years later, a private equity firm by the name of Pegasus Capital Advisors got involved with Carol's Daughter. In exchange for a sizeable financial investment, they became partners in the brand. Carol's Daughter products are now available in Macy's and Sephora stores, on the Home Shopping Network, and even across the pond in the upscale London department store Harrods.

The partnership with Pegasus was crucial for the company's impressive

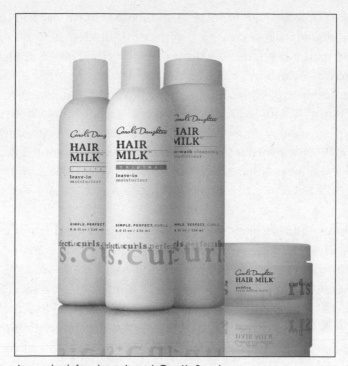

A new look for classic brand Carol's Daughter.
(Courtesy of Carol's Daughter)

expansion—in 2012 Carol's Daughter reportedly earned $35 million in revenues—but the fact that the business no longer belonged solely to Price wasn't broadcast to the masses. After all, who wants to think a group of White men in Connecticut has anything to do with Carol's Daughter products? It just doesn't conjure the same brand image of a business run by a scrappy Black woman with a dream and a nose for success.

Another child of Black hair royalty, Gary Gardner, can relate. Gardner's parents, Edward and Bettiann Gardner, created Soft-Sheen Products Inc. in their family's basement in 1964. That company muscled its way to the top of the Black-owned business world during the seventies and eighties, and Gary took over as president during the company's heyday. But in 1996 Gardner resigned from his position, and two years later Soft Sheen was sold to L'Oréal. But Gary Gardner wasn't finished with the Black hair business. He started his own company, Namaste Laboratories, LLC, the maker of the popular Organic Root Stimulator brand. The Organic Root Stimulator Products—relaxers, conditioners, shampoos, scalp treatments, and more—were sold in

Africa, the Caribbean, and Europe. Many would say Gardner had continued in his parents' footsteps, creating a successful, Black-owned business that capitalized on the booming Black hair industry. However, in 2010, Gardner sold Namaste—which by then commanded 12 percent of the total United States market share of ethnic hair products—in a $100-million cash deal. But his buyer wasn't White or European, or Black. Dabur India Limited, an Indian company looking to enter the Black American and African hair-care market, made Gardner an offer he couldn't refuse. As part of the deal, Gardner maintained his position as CEO at Namaste for an additional five years.

While many in the business world would commend Gardner for a job well done in such a lucrative sale, others, mainly in the Black community, lamented the loss of yet another Black-owned company. Indeed, Black business owners throughout the industry are feeling the pressure. The Black hair salon is seeing encroachment by entrepreneurial Dominicans who have lured Black women away from Black-owned salons with promises of cheaper prices, straighter hair, less chemicals, and shorter wait times. And White-owned salons and brands are jumping on the ethnic hair trend by hiring Black hair experts to work for their companies to up their multicultural cred. (That's what global brand Aveda did in April 2013 when they hired African-American celebrity stylist Tippi Shorter to be their newly created Global Artistic Director of Textured Hair.) The distribution of products at retail is still dominated by Korean storeowners, and the human hair trade, at the export level, is in the hands of the foreign gatekeepers supplying the hair. So, can Black business owners still claim a piece of this very lucrative pie? Quite simply, how do we get back to the good old days?

First it must be recognized that those "good old days" were never that great. While there have always been successful Black hair-care entrepreneurs and industry leaders, White people have always been in the game as well. "We've mythologized a bit what [the majority of Black business owners] were doing in our community," says A'Lelia Bundles, great-great-granddaughter of Madam C. J. Walker, and the biographer of her famous relative. "The reality is we never controlled the market." Bundles admits that while Madam Walker's and Annie Turnbo Malone's hair products were obviously big sellers, "The truth is that in school, in church, and on the bus, the aroma of Dixie Peach and Royal Crown usually was more prevalent than Madam Walker's Hair Conditioning Cream." And by the 2010s, things were not that different. Even though the store shelves were nicely stocked with products made by Black-owned businesses, namely the female hairtrepreneurs making products for natural hair, in the last decade, the top three earners in the mass market ethnic hair category have been L'Oréal USA, Alberto-Culver, and Procter & Gamble.

But what about these enterprising Black women concocting products and taking them to market? They are claiming millions of dollars in sales, but competing against the big guys is another story. "It's really competitive and it's really tough," says Bundles, recalling her childhood growing up with two parents in the hair business. "Today you have to make huge amounts of money to compete with multimillion-dollar corporations. With their deep pockets they can just wait to see what's selling, copy their formula, and then make it cheaper." That's what happened to Wendi Levy and Kim Etheredge, the founders of Mixed Chicks, a company they started in 2004 to address the hair needs of biracial women like themselves. When they were confronted with a copycat these Mixed Chicks fought back. In 2011, when Sally Beauty Supply created a product called Mixed Silk in packaging that looked remarkably like the Mixed Chicks line, Etheredge and Levy sued Sally's and won. A judge required the popular beauty supply company to cease production and sales of Mixed Silk, and they had to pay $8 million in damages to Etheredge and Levy. It's a happy ending for Mixed Chicks, but more imitators are sure to flood the market. And it's debatable whether consumers will buy Black and eschew mainstream products in an act of solidarity. As with all decisions in American commerce, it might not be about Black or White. At the end of the day, the color that matters the most is green.

Obviously, many Black female consumers want to support Black-owned companies when they are looking to buy hair-care products, especially when it comes to products specifically formulated for natural hair, but the reality is that the bigger companies can offer similar products for a much lower price. That was a hard lesson Anu Prestonia of Khamit Kinks learned when she debuted her own line of natural hair products, Anu Essentials, in 2012. "The big boys can charge a lot less for their products because they have the volume that allows them to sell at a lower price point," she says. What's more, Prestonia adds, "They can cut corners and still have a product that performs. They could say they have Moroccan oil in their product and only put one drop of Moroccan oil in there." Jane Carter shares Prestonia's sentiment. "The big guys will either acquire the smaller companies or beat you up in price until you can't compete," she says.

Geri Duncan Jones, fifty-five, is the executive director of the American Health and Beauty Aids Institute, a position she's held since 1988. In her mind, there's no reason to fight over this industry. Even though her organization exists to support Black-owned businesses in the ethnic beauty industry, she's not worrying about a takeover. "There is an opportunity for everyone in the manufacturing and distribution channel to be successful," Jones says. "Black business owners who are business savvy are not threatened by other distributors or manufacturers." Carter puts her own spin on this idea. "I think the real visionaries will have staying power because they have really created value for their customers," she says. "The ones who've put a lifetime into this business will be fine."

The Black Hair Industry Gets De-Racialized

Anthony Dickey of Hair Rules knows and has known that the future of hair care is about texture, not race. "At the end of the day, race is the reason we have this problematic 'one size fits all' approach to hair care," says Dickey, lambasting this industry that assumes all Black people have the same hair type, or all White people do for that matter. He urges salons and product manufacturers to make products for all textures and likewise, retail outlets to stock products for all textures. That's what he's done with his Hair Rules salon and product line. Even though his message of embracing one's natural tresses resonates strongly with Black women, the clientele in his salon and the customers who buy his products run the gamut. According to his own company research, one-third of the customers who buy his products are White. At his New York City salon, Dickey estimates, 80 percent of his clients are Black. But on any given day, it "looks like a Benetton commercial," he says.

Ironically, that's how things ended in the last century. John Paul DeJoria from John Paul Mitchell Systems predicted the future of hair care was going to be about texture, not race. And he clearly put his money where his mouth is, because DeJoria invested in and joined the board of Texture-Media, the Web-based company that owns NaturallyCurly.com and CurlyNikki.com as well as the very profitable e-commerce site CurlMart

.com. The CEO of TextureMedia is a White woman with straight hair, but that doesn't mean she can't cater to the needs of the 2.5 million diverse, curly-haired women who spend $1 billion annually on hair products, which is what TextureMedia does. "We're an equal-opportunity company," laughs TextureMedia President and Naturally Curly.com cofounder Michelle Breyer, who is also White, but has curly hair. Breyer knows that Black women and White women have different experiences when it comes to their curly hair, but that's not what the company focuses on. "I think we have more in common than many people believe," she says. "Our struggles are very similar when it comes to self-image and the unpredictability of our hair." As such, TextureMedia is harnessing the spending power of their 2.5 million users and making money from advertising, product sales, and selling market research. And as for those who want to continue to segment the hair-care industry by race, Breyer thinks they will go the way of the dinosaur.

Lisa Price of Carol's Daughter agrees. "You can't put a label on what is Black hair. There's no such thing as 'Black hair,' just like there isn't one single type of White hair," she says, adding that with the growing numbers of multiracial Americans, the idea of a race-based hair industry is a useless paradigm. "What we're really dealing with is textured hair," Price insists. Even at her Harlem-based salon Mirrors, where Price attracts mostly African-American women, she firmly declares, "We embrace everyone, and all textures are welcome."

From a business perspective, people like Lisa Price, Jane Carter, and Anthony Dickey appear to be on the path for continued success. And there are plenty of non-Black hair-care entrepreneurs on the textured track who have garnered a loyal, multiracial following as well. Salons like Devachan and Ouidad were created for curlies but not for any particular race (and they both have successful product lines, too). So it seems that anybody who can style "textured" hair, make products for "textured hair," write about "textured hair," throw parties for "textured hair" or build a Web site about "textured hair" can ride that ride all the way to the bank.

"The hair-care industry will evolve because the changing U.S. demographic will force it to," says Jane Carter. Perhaps by 2043, when demographers predict the U.S. population will no longer be a White majority, the ethnic hair-care industry will simply cease to exist. From then on it will simply be recognized as mainstream. Regardless of what we call it, however, it seems clear that Black hair will always mean big business.

Top 10 New Millennium Moments in Black Hair History

2000: In time for the release of her second album, singer Erykah Badu unwinds her nearly mile-high head wrap and reveals a head full of long locs underneath. Turns out they weren't her actual hair but extensions. Badu, who later would wear Afro wigs, straight weaves, and even a blond blunt-cut wig, saw it as nobody's business but her own how she wore her hair—though many fans felt it was blasphemous for the super-spiritual Badu to fake the style. In response Badu said, "This hair don't make me," proving it less than a year later when she shaved her head bald.

2001: Historically Black institution Hampton University prohibits male MBA students from having cornrows or locs. Dean of the Business School Sid Credle says he wants the men to look professional so they can get jobs. He also defends his decision, saying, "When was it that cornrows and dredlocs were a part of African-American history? I mean Charles Drew didn't wear it, Muhammad Ali didn't wear it, Martin Luther King didn't wear it."

2002: The movie *Barbershop,* starring Ice Cube and Cedric the Entertainer, grabs the number-one spot at the box office during its opening weekend and goes on to gross more than $75 million. The unexpected crossover hit set mostly in a Black barbershop spawns a sequel, *Barbershop 2,* and a spin-off, *Beautyshop,* starring Queen Latifah.

2005: Biracial *New Yorker* staff writer Malcolm Gladwell gets in on the hair conversation in his bestselling book *Blink,* detailing how he began getting stopped routinely by police for traffic violations and pulled out of line by the TSA at airports after growing his hair into an Afro. "Even though I was exactly the same person, once I had longer hair the world saw me as being profoundly different," he told CNN.

2006: The Brazilian keratin treatment (BKT) is introduced to the American market with promises of providing semipermanent straight hair without harsh chemicals. Most consumers are unaware that the BKT was discovered by a Brazilian mortician who realized that formalde-hyde was straightening the hair of his corpses. As such, formaldehyde is the main ingredient in the BKT. Neither the ick factor, nor the fact that formaldehyde is a known carcinogen, stems the flow of women lining up for the expensive treatment.

2009: Disney debuts its first African-American princess, Princess Tiana, in the film *The Princess and the Frog* and teams up with Carol's Daughter to create a Princess Tiana line of hair and bath products. The shampoo, conditioner, detangler, and bubble bath were said to be "beauty staples Princess Tiana would most likely use," effectively making them the first Disney products made with Black girls in mind.

2010: Miss Jessie's hair products debut at Target stores nationwide. This is a coup not only for Miss Jessie's founders, but also for all the curly girls around the country who wanted to try their luscious-sounding products. It's not until March 2012, however, that Target makes Black hair history by desegregating their hair aisles and moving the Miss Jessie's products to the now integrated professional hair-care shelves.

2011: Rihanna famously responds to Twitter follower NinyaBella, a woman who tweeted the pop singer when she saw Rih Rih's new photo, "Why does her hair look so nappy?" Rihanna's answer: "Because I'm Black, bitch."

2012: Oprah appears on the cover of her magazine *O* with unstraightened hair in an issue themed around makeovers and transformations. Though Winfrey says she often wears her hair this way off-camera, she also admits that she once "wanted to wear it close-cropped à la Camille Cosby but Camille's husband, Bill, convinced me otherwise. 'Don't do it,' he said. 'You've got the wrong head shape and you'll disappoint yourself.'" She took his advice—and was back to straight and bouncy for the next month's cover.

Sources

CHAPTER 1

Barbot, Jean. *Barbot on Guinea: The Writings of Jean Barbot on West Africa, 1678–1712*. Edited by P.E.H. Hair. Hakluyt Society, 1992.

Boone, Sylvia Ardyn. *Radiance from the Waters: Ideals of Feminine Beauty in Mende Art*. New Haven: Yale University Press, 1986.

Curtin, Philip D., ed. *Africa Remembered: Narratives by West Africans from the Era of the Slave Trade*. Madison: University of Wisconsin Press, 1967.

Davidson, Basil. *The African Slave Trade*. Boston: Little, Brown, 1961.

Estell, Kenneth. *African America: Portrait of a People*. Farmington Hills, Mich.: Visible Ink Press, 1993.

Gatewood, Willard B. *Aristocrats of Color: The Black Elite, 1880–1920*. Bloomington: Indiana University Press, 1990.

Hodges, Graham Russell, and Alan Edward Brown, eds. *Pretends to Be Free: Runaway Slave Advertisements from Colonial and Revolutionary New York and New Jersey*. New York: Garland, 1994.

Hogg, Peter C. *Slavery, the Afro-American Experience*. London: British Library, 1979.

Johnson, Charles, and Patricia Smith. *Africans in America: America's Journey Through Slavery*. San Diego: Harcourt Brace, 1998.

Lincoln, C. Eric, and Lawrence H. Mamiya. *The Black Church in the African American Experience*. Durham, N.C.: Duke University Press, 1990.

Meaders, Daniel, ed. *Advertisements for Runaway Slaves in Virginia, 1801–1820*. New York: Garland, 1997.

Mellon, James. *Bullwhip Days: The Slaves Remember*. New York: Avon, 1988.

Molnar, Stephen. *Human Variation: Races, Types, and Ethnic Groups*. Englewood Cliffs, N.J.: Prentice Hall, 1975.

Morrow, Willie L. *400 Years Without a Comb*. San Diego: Black Publishers of San Diego, 1973.

Ogunwale, Titus. *African Traditional Hairdos*. Ife-Ife, Nigeria: Kosalabaro Press, 1976.

Piersen, William D. *From Africa to America: African American History from the Colonial Era to the Early Republic, 1526–1790*. New York: Twayne, 1996.

Sterling, Dorothy, and Mary Helen Washington. *We Are Your Sisters*. New York: Norton, 1984.

White, Shane, and Graham J. White. *Stylin': African-American Expressive Culture from Its Beginnings to the Zoot Suit*. Ithaca: Cornell University Press, 1998.

Williamson, Joel. *New People: Miscegenation and Mulattoes in the United States*. Baton Rouge: Louisiana State University Press, 1995.

CHAPTER 2

Boston, Lloyd. *Men of Color: Fashion, History, Fundamentals*. New York: Artisan, 1998.

Bundles, A'Lelia Perry. *Madam C. J. Walker*. New York: Chelsea House Publishers, 1991.

Due, Tananarive. *The Black Rose*. New York: One World/Random House, 2000.

Gates, Henry Louis. "Madam's Crusade." *Time*, December 7, 1998.

Giddings, Paula. *When and Where I Enter: The Impact of Black Women on Race and Sex in America*. New York: William Morrow, 1996.

Graham, Lawrence Otis. *Our Kind of People: Inside America's Black Upper Class*. New York: HarperCollins, 1999.

"Hair Attachments," *Ebony*, June 1947.

Hall, Ronald, Kathy Russell, and Midge Wilson. *Color Complex: The Politics of Skin Color Among African-Americans*. New York: Anchor Books/Doubleday, 1992.

Kelley, Robin D. G. "Nap Time: Historicizing the Afro." *Fashion Theory* 1(4), 1997.

Larsen, Nella. *Quicksand and Passing*. American Women Writers Series. Piscataway, N.J.: Rutgers University Press, 1986.

Locke, Alain L. *The New Negro: An Interpretation*. New York: A. and C. Boni, 1925.

Lynk, B. S. *A Complete Course in Hair Straightening and Beauty Culture*. Memphis, Tenn.: 20th Century Art Co., 1919.

Madam C. J. Walker Archives, Indiana Historical Society.

Ottley, Roi. "5 Million U.S. White Negroes," *Ebony*, March 1948.

Peiss, Kathy. *Hope in a Jar: The Making of America's Beauty Culture*. New York: Henry Holt, 1998.

Rooks, Noliwe. *Hair Raising: Beauty, Culture, and African American Women*. Piscataway, N.J.: Rutgers University Press, 1996.

Smith, Jessie Carney, ed. "Annie Turnbo Malone." In *Notable Black American Women*. Farmington Hills, Mich: Gale Group, 1992.

Thurman, Wallace. *The Blacker the Berry*. New York: Arno Press, 1969.

Walker, Juliet E. K. *The History of Black Business in America: Capitalism, Race, Entrepreneurship*. New York: Twayne, 1998.

White, Graham, and Shane White. *Stylin': African-American Expressive Culture from Its Beginnings to the Zoot Suit*. Ithaca: Cornell University Press, 1998.

X, Malcolm, and Alex Haley. *The Autobiography of Malcolm X*. New York: Grove Press, 1965.

CHAPTER 3

Boston, Lloyd. *Men of Color: Fashion, History, Fundamentals*. New York: Artisan, 1998.

Campbell, Lorna. "Great Moments in Hair." *Washingtonian Magazine*, August 1998.

Duke, Sharon. "Afro Horizons." *Ethnic Newswatch*, August 31, 1994.

Hamilton, Charles V. "How Black Is Black?" *Ebony*, August 1969.

Kelley, Robin D. G. "Nap Time: Historicizing the Afro." *Fashion Theory* 1(4), 1997.

Jones, Lois Liberty, and John Henry Jones. *All About the Natural*. Clairol Books, 1971.

Milloy, Courtland T. "The Afro Doing a Graceful Fadeout." *Washington Post*, June 27, 1977.

Morris, Bernadine. "Hair-Cuts: Hair Stylist Is Honored by Blacks He Inspired." *New York Times*, June 25, 1980.

Morrow, Willie L. *400 Years Without a Comb*. San Diego: Black Publishers of San Diego, 1973.

Nelson, Jill. "Enough to Curl Your Hair." *Washington Post*, December 6, 1987.

———. *Straight, No Chaser: How I Became a Grown-Up Black Woman*. New York: Penguin Putnam, 1997.

Peacock, Mary. "10 Haircuts That Shook the World." *InStyle*, March 1997.

Shakur, Assata. *Assata: An Autobiography*. Chicago: Lawrence Hill Books, 1988.

Simone, Nina. *I Put a Spell on You: The Autobiography of Nina Simone*. New York: Da Capo Press, 1993.

Walker, Juliet E. K. *The History of Black Business in America: Capitalism, Race, Entrepreneurship*. New York: Twayne, 1998.

CHAPTER 4

Bray, Rosemary. "Reclaiming Our Culture." *Essence*, December 1990.

Bundles, A'Lelia Perry. *Madam C. J. Walker*. New York: Chelsea House, 1991.

Canedy, Dana. "The Courtship of Black Consumers." *New York Times*, August 11, 1998.

Colwell, Shelly M. "Lasting Locs: Targeting the Ethnic Hair Market." *Soap Cosmetics Chemical Specialties*, May 1996.

Day, Sherri. "The Economics of Hair." *East Bay Express*, June 16, 2000.

Feder, Barnaby J. "A Leader in Black Business, Johnson Products to Be Sold." *New York Times*, June 15, 1993.

Gates, Henry Louis. "Madam's Crusade." *Time*, December 7, 1998.

Gatewood, Willard B. *Aristocrats of Color: The Black Elite, 1880–1920*. Bloomington: Indiana University Press, 1990.

"Help for Blacks Has Roots in Hair Care." *Canadian Press Newswire*, June 9, 1996.

Jones, Lisa. *Bulletproof Diva: Tales of Race, Sex and Hair*. New York: Doubleday, 1994.

Lyon, Paula. "For the Record." *Crain's Chicago Business*, June 22, 1998.

Margot, Raven. "Minority Merchandising: Building a Loyal Base." *Drug Topics*, May 7, 1984.

McCaffery, Jen. "Rapunzel's Offspring Are Cashing In." *New York Times*, February 20, 2000.

Morrow, Willie L. *400 Years Without a Comb*. San Diego: Black Publishers of San Diego, 1973.

"New Hair Culture Discovery: Mexican Chemist Claims Process to Make Negro Hair Straight, Silky," *Ebony*, June 1948.

Parks, Liz. "Despite Tough Ethnic Market, Hair Color, Relaxers Score Double Digit Gains." *Drug Store News*, April 1, 1996.

Peiss, Kathy. *Hope in a Jar: The Making of America's Beauty Culture*. New York: Henry Holt, 1998.

Poe, Janita. "Parting Ways." *Chicago Tribune*, August 23, 1993.

Pulley, Bret. "Profit Over Pride." *Emerge*, January 31, 1994.

Rooks, Noliwe M. *Hair Raising: Beauty, Culture, and African American Women*. Piscataway, N.J.: Rutgers University Press, 1996.

Syed, Ali N. "Ethnic Hair Care: History, Trends and Formulations." *Cosmetics and Toiletries*, September 1993.

Walker, Juliet E. K. *The History of Black Business in America: Capitalism, Race, Entrepreneurship*, New York: Twayne, 1998.

Wang, Malone, and Maggie Malone. "Can Revlon Repair Its Image?" *Newsweek*, February 23, 1987.

———. "Targeting Black Dollars." *Newsweek*, October 13, 1986.

White, Shane, and Graham J. White. *Stylin': African-American Expressive Culture from Its Beginnings to the Zoot Suit.* Ithaca, N.Y.: Cornell University Press, 1998.

CHAPTER 5

Anate, Isa. "Locked Out?" *Essence*, August 1990.

"The Artistry of African-Inspired Braids." *New York Times*, September 8, 1991.

Blankson, Naadu I. "The Dreaded Decision." *Essence*, May 1990.

"Bo Derek." *E! True Hollywood Story*, 1999.

Bordo, Susan. *Unbearable Weight: Feminism, Western Culture, and the Body.* Berkeley: University of California Press, 1993.

"Bo's Braids." *Newsweek*, January 28, 1980.

Boston, Lloyd. *Men of Color: Fashion, History, Fundamentals.* New York: Artisan, 1998.

Bowden, Mark. "Survivor of MOVE Disaster Still Haunted." *Times-Picayune*, May 14, 1995.

"The Braided Bunch." *Newsweek*, January 28, 1980.

Britt, Donna. "Short Cuts and Head Lines." *Washington Post*, October 22, 1989.

Chevannes, Barry. *Rastafari: Roots and Ideology.* Syracuse, N.Y.: Syracuse University Press, 1994.

"Corporate Dress Codes Can Turn Hair-Raising." *Chicago Tribune*, March 28, 1988.

Davis, Angela. "Afro Images: Politics, Fashion and Nostalgia." In *The Angela Y. Davis Reader*, edited by Joy James. Malden, Mass.: Blackwell Publishers, 1988.

DuCille, Ann. *Skin Trade.* Cambridge: Harvard University Press, 1996.

Dunbar, Donnette. "Only Her Hairdresser Knows . . . ," *Omaha World-Herald*, August 19, 1997.

Duncombe, Ted. "Ten Years Later, MOVE Inferno Still Burns in Memories." Associated Press, May 7, 1995.

Gilliam, Dorothy. "Cornrows Don't Belong to Bo." *Washington Post*, February 4, 1980.

Gregory, Deborah. "They Shoot Models, Don't They?" *Essence*, April 1991.

"The Hair Wars." *InStyle*, October 1999.

Henderson, Greg. "Marriott Called Discriminatory in Cornrow Case." United Press International, April 27, 1988.

Hines, Tanya M. "To Weave or Not to Weave?" *Philadelphia Tribune*, October 26, 1993.

"Hotel Allows Clerk to Keep Ethnic Hairstyle." *Washington Dateline*, January 7, 1988.

Jones, Lisa. *Bulletproof Diva: Tales of Race, Sex and Hair.* New York: Doubleday, 1994.

Kern-Foxworth, Marilyn. "Plantation Kitchen to American Icon: Aunt Jemima, Publicity, and American Culture." *Public Relations Review*, September 2, 1990.

Key, Janet. "At Age 100, a New Aunt Jemima." *Chicago Tribune*, April 28, 1989.

Kirby, Marilyn. "Stylish Young Black Men are Looking Sharp in Angled Haircuts." *Orange County (New Jersey) Register*, June 2 1989.

Leff, Lisa. "Getting a Loc on the Look Isn't Easy." *Washington Post*, December 7, 1994.

Leiter, Robert. "Burning Down the House: MOVE and the Tragedy in Philadelphia." *New Leader*, September 21, 1987.

Marriott, Michel. "Colorstuck." *Essence*, November 1991.

Martin, Lois Mufuka. "African-American Women Facing Tough Road with Corporate America over Hairstyles." *New Pittsburgh Courier*, July 17, 1993.

Mastalia, Francesco, and Alfonse Pagano. *Dreads*. New York: Artisan, 1999.

McLaughlin, Patricia. "There's a Twisted Logic Behind a Fear of Braids." *St. Louis Post-Dispatch*, October 28, 1993.

Mercer, Kobena. "Black Hair/Style Politics." In *Out There: Marginalization and Contemporary Cultures*, edited by Russell Ferguson, Martha Gever, Trinh T. Minh-ha, and Cornel West. Cambridge: MIT Press, 1992.

"Michael Jackson's Doctor Credits Nurse for First Aid." *San Diego Union-Tribune*, February 3, 1984.

Nicholas, Tracy. *Rastafari: A Way of Life*. New York: Anchor Books, 1979.

Paul, Jim. "Cafeteria Refuses to Rehire Worker with Do, Despite ACLU Complaint." Associated Press, April 19, 1988.

Perry, Tony. "San Diego at Large: She's Head-to-Head with LaCosta in a Hairy, Tangled Labor Dispute." *Los Angeles Times*, October 30, 1991.

"Reviews from the Hairstyle Critics." *Washington Post*, October 22, 1989.

Rose, Tricia. *Black Noise: Rap Music and Black Culture in Contemporary America*. Hanover, N.H.: University Press of New England, 1994.

Ruffins, Paul. "Hair to the Throne." *Washington City Paper*, January 15, 1999.

Sajbel, Maureen. "Coming Up with a Fast Fade." *Los Angeles Times*, September 11, 1991.

Schachter, Jim. "EEOC Says Hyatt Showed Bias in Its Ban on Cornrows." *Los Angeles Times*, May 17, 1988.

Sharpton, Al. *Go and Tell Pharoah: The Autobiography of the Reverend Al Sharpton*. New York: Doubleday, 1996.

Shipp, E. R. "Are Cornrows Right for Work?" *Essence*, February 1988.

———. "Braided Hair Style at Issue in Protests Over Dress Codes." *New York Times*, September 23, 1987.

"Singer Leaves Hospital After Hair Catches Fire." *New York Times*, January 29, 1984.

"Sisters Love the Weave." *Essence*, August 1990.

Sweeney, Louise. "A Viola in her Voice." *Christian Science Monitor*, March 6, 1980.

Zausner, Robert. "Scars, Questions Remain a Year After MOVE Battle." United Press International, May 11, 1986.

Zoglin, Richard. "Too Much Risk on the Set?" *Time*, February 13, 1984.

"9-to-5 Braids." *Essence*, May 1988.

CHAPTER 6

Bonner, Lonnice Brittenum. *Good Hair: For Colored Girls Who've Considered Weaves When the Chemicals Became Too Ruff.* New York: Crown, 1994.

Bordo, Susan. *Unbearable Weight: Feminism, Western Culture, and the Body.* Berkeley: University of California Press, 1993.

Bray, Rosemary. "Reclaiming Our Culture." *Essence,* December 1990.

Collins, Patricia Hill. *Black Feminist Thought: Knowledge, Consciousness, and the Politics of Empowerment.* New York: Routledge, 1990.

DuCille, Ann. *Skin Trade.* Cambridge: Harvard University Press, 1996.

"The Ebony Advisor." *Ebony,* January 2000.

Gregory, Deborah. "They Shoot Models Don't They?" *Essence,* April 1991.

hooks, bell. *Black Looks: Race and Representation.* Cambridge, Mass.: South End Press, 1992.

———. *Bone Black: Memories of Girlhood.* New York: Henry Holt, 1996.

Jones, Lisa. *Bulletproof Diva: Tales of Race, Sex and Hair.* New York: Doubleday, 1994.

Jurmain, Robert, Harry Nelson, Lynn Kilgore, and Wenda Trevathan. *Introduction to Physical Anthropology.* Belmont, Calif.: Wadsworth, 2000.

Lee, Felicia R. "Blond Ambition in the Urban Mosaic." *New York Times,* October 10, 1999.

Mancuso, Kevin. *The Mane Thing.* Boston: Little, Brown, 1999.

Marriott, Michael. "Colorstruck." *Essence,* November 1991.

Mcdowell, Akkida. "The Art of the Ponytail." In *Adiós, Barbie: Young Women Write about Body Image and Identity,* edited by Ophira Edut. Seattle: Seal Press, 1998.

Mercer, Kobena. "Black Hair/Style Politics." In *Out There: Marginalization and Contemporary Culture,* edited by Russel Feruson, Martha Gever, Trinh T. Minh-ha, and Cornell West. Cambridge: MIT Press, 1992.

Nelson, Jill. *Straight, No Chaser: How I Became a Grown-Up Black Woman.* New York: Penguin Putnam, 1997.

Rooks, Noliwe M. *Hair Raising: Beauty, Culture, and African American Women.* Piscataway, N.J.: Rutgers University Press, 1996.

Russell, Kathy Y., Midge Wilson, and Ronald Hall. *The Color Complex: The Politics of Skin Color Among African Americans.* New York: Anchor Books, 1992.

Sieber, Roy. *Hair in African Art and Culture: Status, Symbol and Style.* Munich, Germany: Prestel Verlag, 2000.

Simons, Janet. "Love Is Color Blind." *Denver Rocky Mountain News,* February 7, 1999.

Washington, Elsie B. "Nothing Fake." *Essence,* November 1991.

Wilson, Midge, and Kathy Russell. *Divided Sisters: Bridging the Gap Between Black Women and White Women.* New York: Anchor Books, 1996.

CHAPTER 7

Chambers, Veronica. "Blond Like Me." *New York Times*, June 25, 1995.

Davis, Peter. "Good Head: Hot Irons." *Paper*, May 1999.

"Hair Today, Hair Tomorrow." *Ebony*, May 1998.

Herron, Carolivia. *Nappy Hair*. New York: Knopf, 1997.

hooks, bell. *Happy to Be Nappy*. New York: Hyperion, 1999.

Horyn, Cathy. "Go with the Fro." *Washington Post*, March 15, 1994.

Johnson, Adrienne M. "Do or Dye." *Los Angeles Times*, June 8, 1995.

Jones, Linda. "Author Surprised by Controversy Book Sparked." *Dallas Morning News*, June 16, 1999.

———. "Nappy Hair." *Greensboro News & Record*, January 9, 1999.

Jones, Sabrina. "Dance Is Over, but Talk Goes On." *Raleigh News & Observer*, February 18, 1999.

Lee, Felicia R. "Blond Ambition in the Urban Mosaic." *New York Times*, October 10, 1999.

Martin, Michelle H. "Never Too Nappy." *Horn Book Magazine*, May 1, 1999.

McDowell, Akkida. "The Art of the Ponytail." In *Adiós, Barbie: Young Women Write about Body Image and Identity*, edited by Ophira Edut. Seattle: Seal Press, 1998.

Merida, Kevin. "The Bush Doctor Is Very In." *Washington Post*, April 30, 1999.

Meyer, Lisa. "National Perspective: Update: 'Nappy Hair' Still Touchy Class Subject." *Los Angeles Times*, March 25, 1999.

Mitchell, Mary. "Banning Hairstyles Cheat Students of Lesson on Culture." *Chicago Sun-Times*, November 10, 1996.

"Modern Living." *Time*, December 24, 1973.

Ogunnaike, Lola. "Some Hair Is Happy to Be Nappy." *New York Times*, December 27, 1998.

Oppel, Shelby. "Third Graders Braided Hair Sparks Cultural Dispute." *St. Petersburg Times*, December 9, 1996.

Ruffins, Paul. "Hair to the Throne." *Washington City Paper*, January 15, 1999.

Schjeldahl, Peter. "The Nasty Brits: How Sensational Is 'Sensation?'" *New Yorker*, October 11, 1999.

"Sunday Forum." *Raleigh News & Observer*, November 22, 1998.

Terrell, Angela. "The Bush Doctor." *Washington Post*, May 30, 1971.

CHAPTER 8

"Your Race, Your Looks." *Glamour*. February 2008.

Andrews, Jessica. "How Natural is Too Natural?" *New York Times*. June 25, 2012.

Bey, Jamila. "Going Natural Requires Lots of Help." *New York Times*, June 8, 2011.

Blay, Yaba. *(1)ne Drop: Shifting the Lens on Race*. Philadelphia: Blackprint Press, 2014.

Byrd, Ayana. "Headsprung." *Vibe Vixen*, Spring 2005.

Carter, Ernessa T. and Walton, Nikki. *Better Than Good Hair*. New York: Amistad, 2013.

DaCosta, Diane. *Textured Tresses: The Ultimate Guide to Maintaining and Styling Natural Hair*. New York: Touchstone, 2004.

Hajela, Deepti. "Don Imus' 'Nappy' Remark Has Long, Hurtful History in Describing African-American Hair." *Associated Press*. April 12, 2007.

Holmes, Tamara E. "Natural Hair is Big Business." *Black Enterprise*, January/February 2013.

Lucas, Demetria L. "Why Does My Natural Hair Get No Love?" *The Root*, September 20, 2012.

Millner, Denene. "Blue Ivy's Hair: Seriously, Folk—Leave Beyoncé and Jay Z's Child All the Way Alone Already." *My Brown Baby*, May 1, 2013.

Moe. "'Glamour' Editor to Lady Lawyers: Apparently Being Black is Kinda a Corporate 'Don't.'" *Jezebel.com*, August 14, 2007.

NPR Staff. "'I Love My Hair': A Father's Tribute to His Daughter." NPR, October 18, 2010.

Pitt, Brad. "My List." *Esquire*, October 2006.

Puente, Maria. "Chris Rock's 'Good Hair' Gets Tangled Up in Controversy." *USA Today*, October 25, 2009.

Saint Louis, Catherine. "Black Hair, Still Tangled in Politics." *New York Times*, August 26, 2009.

Samuels, Allison. "Gabby Douglas Takes Two Olympic Golds—And Hair Criticism." *The Daily Beast*. August 2, 2012.

Samuels, Allison. "Zahara Jolie-Pitt and the Politics of Uncombed Hair." *The Daily Beast*. October 9, 2009.

Sangweni, Yolanda. "Meteorologist Rhonda Lee on Getting Fired, Being Labeled the Rosa Parks of Natural Hair." *Essence.com*. January 10, 2013.

Stewart, Dodai. "How Does a Black Women Feel About the *Glamour* Controversy? I Asked Myself!" *Jezebel.com*. October 9, 2007.

Valdés, Mimi. "Simply Irresistible." *Vibe*. September 2002.

Walker, Brittney M. "Gabby Douglas Gets a Famous Hairstylist." *EUR Web*. August 16, 2012.

Wheat, Alynda. "Good Hair? Hardly. How Chris Rock Got it Wrong." *Entertainment Weekly*. October 12, 2009.

Wiltz, Teresa. "'Good Hair,' Bad Vibes." *The Root*. October 8, 2009.

Wilkerson, Isabel. "Gabrielle Douglas Responds to Hair Criticism: 'What's Wrong With My Hair?'" *The Daily Beast*. August 6, 2012.

Yursik, Patrice. "Tyra Banks Real Hair Dismay." *Afrobella*. September 9, 2009.

Chapter 9

Beard, Hilary and Lisa Price. *Success Never Smelled So Sweet: How I Followed My Nose and Found My Passion*. New York: One World/Ballantine, 2004.

Bey, Jamila. "Going Natural Requires Lots of Help." *New York Times*, June 8, 2011.

Boyle, A. F. "Entrepreneurs Reclaim Black Hair Care Market from White Firms." *Associated Press*, March 1, 2008.

Carney, Scott. "The Temple of Do." *Mother Jones*, March/April 2010.

Dade, Corey. "Much Ado About Straightening: Old Black Salons Face New Rivals." *Wall Street Journal*, May 12, 2010.

Grubow, Liz, and Elle Morris. "The Imperative Relevance of Ethnic Hair Care." *Global Cosmetic Industry Magazine*, July 2010.

Holmes, Tamara E. "Natural Hair is Big Business." *Black Enterprise*, January/February 2013.

Hyde, Marina. "A Rough Cut." *The Guardian*, February 12, 2004.

Khaleeli, Homa. "The Hair Trade's Dirty Secret." *The Guardian*, October 28, 2012.

Kinosian, Janet. "Beauty Products Made with Natural Ingredients." *Los Angeles Times*, April 22, 2012.

Mamgain, Pramugdha. "Dabur Buys US Hair Care Co. for $100mn." *The Economic Times*, November 16, 2010.

Montague-Jones, Guy. "P&G Sells African-American Hair Care Business." *Cosmetics Design.com*, April 1, 2009.

Pettigrew, Mika. "Taking Back the Black Hair Care Industry." *Clutch Magazine*, April 1, 2007.

Robb, Amanda. "She Got Rich Doing What?!" *More Magazine*. July/August 2013.

Ross, Janell. "Natural or Relaxed, For Black Women, Hair Is Not a Settled Matter." *Huffington Post BlackVoices*, August 04, 2011.

Tavernise, Sabrina. "A Thriving Growth Area in a Weak Economy: Hair." *New York Times*, August 6, 2011.

Wellington, Elizabeth. "Hair Together." *Philadelphia Inquirer*, November 3, 2010.

Williams, Tia. "Ask the Experts: Brazilian Keratin Treatment." *Essence.com*, March 4, 2010.

Williams, Timothy. "Costly Hairstyle Is a Beauty Trend That Draws Thieves' Notice." *New York Times*, May 1, 2011.

Wilson, Ni'kita. "Johnson Products Back in Black Hands." *The Grio.com*. July 16, 2009.

Index